the new beauty secrets

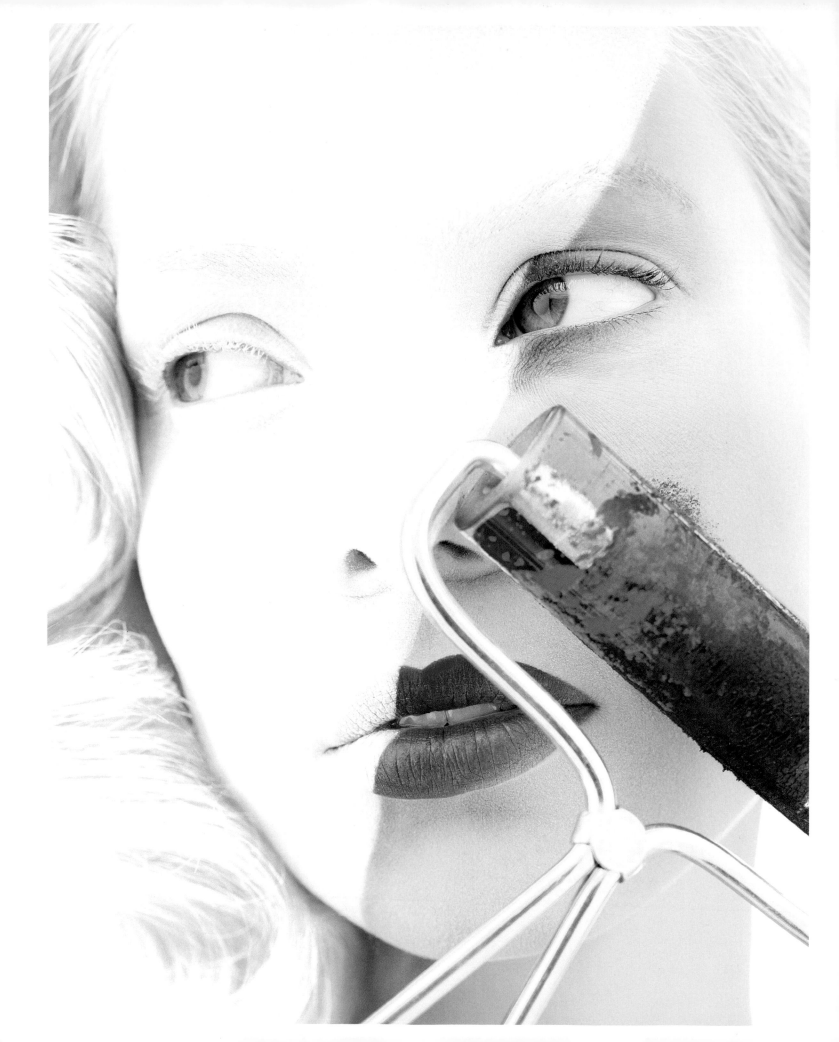

the new beauty secrets

Your Ultimate Guide to a Flawless Face

Laura Mercier

Makeup by Laura Mercier

Still Life Photography by Richard Pierce

Cover and Illustrations by Izak

Creative Direction by Ranee Flynn

Art Direction by Julian Peploe

Photo Research by Sandra Collado

Atria Books

New York   London   Toronto   Sydney

Photo by Raymond Meier

For Danielle Rouille

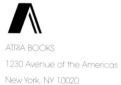

ATRIA BOOKS
1230 Avenue of the Americas
New York, NY 10020

Library of Congress Cataloging-in-Publication Data

ISBN-13: 978-0-7432-9631-1
ISBN-10: 0-7432-9631-1

First Atria Books hardcover edition October 2006

10 9 8 7 6 5 4 3 2 1

ATRIA B O O K S is a trademark of Simon & Schuster, Inc.

Manufactured in the United States of America

For information about special discounts for bulk purchases, please contact Simon & Schuster Special
Sales at 1-800-456-6798 or business@simonandschuster.com.

Madonna by Patrick Demarchelier

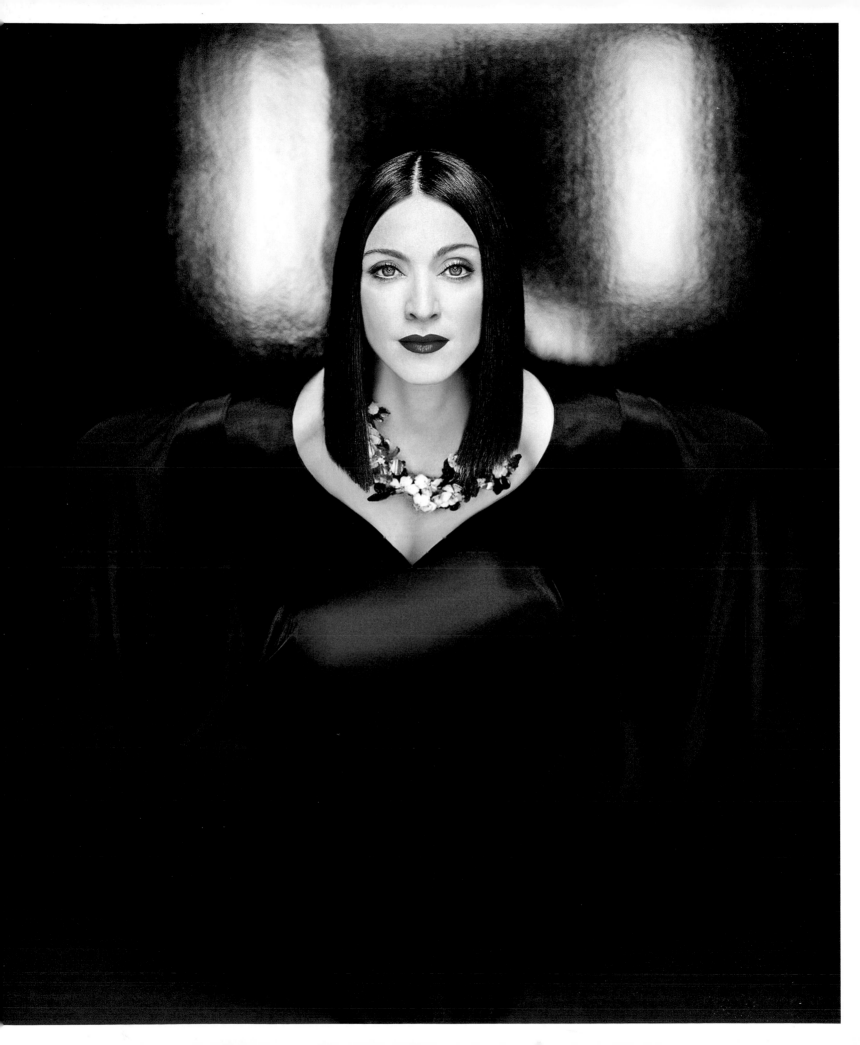

This book is dedicated to those who delight in

bringing beauty into their lives and the lives of others

contents

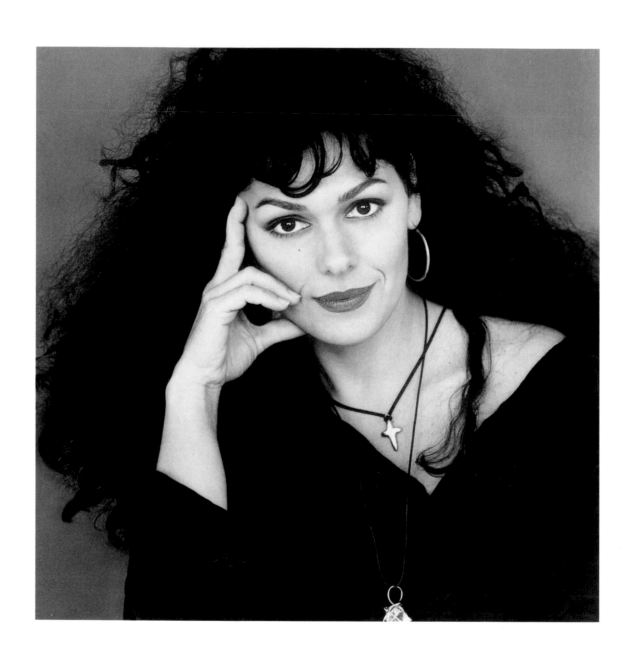

introduction

It took me a long time to accept the idea of doing a book. I thought everything had been said and done, and no one would want to hear more about lipstick, eyeliner, and blush. What convinced me was the realization that I could go beyond the tricks and tips of my profession to help others see beauty with a slightly different eye—with a more gentle, indulgent eye, in fact. You'll certainly learn how to achieve the best application of makeup possible from the pages ahead; but there is a deeper journey you may want to take and that is to start looking at yourself differently. It took me fifteen years to make peace with the woman I was seeing in the mirror. I know today that appreciating your own beauty does not come solely from therapy, makeup application, or plastic surgery—although these things can help. Rather, it comes from a little door that opens in our minds and helps us celebrate our differences and find pride in our uniqueness. As my friend Peter says, "There is only one of you!" If you don't realize this, I hope I can teach you to see it for yourself.

—Laura Mercier

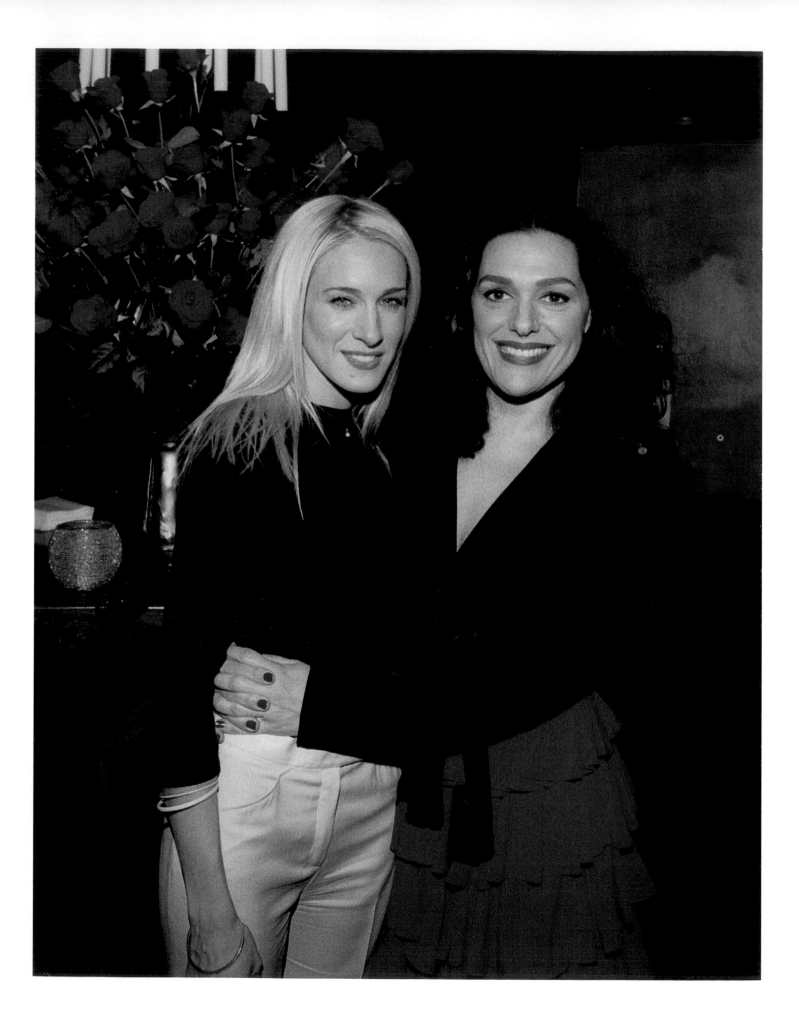

foreword

When you do many photo shoots, you pay attention to pictures in magazines or taken at red carpet appearances. Years ago, any time I thought an actress looked good, I always checked the makeup credits, and there was one name that came up time and time again—Laura Mercier. I pursued her for years, and we finally got to work together for a *Marie Claire* cover with photographer Patrick Demarchelier. There was something different about Laura. Any decent makeup artist can make an eighteen-year-old look amazing, but Laura can also make a woman look amazing. Believe it or not, that makes her unique in her field. She understands the difference between makeup for a girl and makeup for a woman. Perhaps it has to do with the fact that Laura is a completely natural, beautiful woman who doesn't believe in clinging to her youth. She believes this so strongly that today's fountains of youth actually offend her aesthetic. She is truly interested in women's faces with all their perfections and imperfections. She understands how faces change and how certain muscles move, making us laugh, smile, or frown. It's as if she has studied film clips of facial expressions and memorized how the interplay of shadow and light can alter and reveal so much. In fact, she's more like a painter or a physiologist than a makeup artist.

Another thing about Laura is her sense of elegance and taste. She has a wonderful European aesthetic because she spent her most influential years in the South of France and in Paris. That dark, mysterious mouth that French women carry so well is a favorite look of hers, and she always wants to do it on me. I'm afraid of color because I think it makes my mouth seem tiny, so we battle it out. Every color looks good on Laura because she has these gorgeous big lips, and she's much more of a risk taker in that

Sarah Jessica and Laura by Silvia Mautner

area than I am. On *Sex and the City*, I didn't wear any lipstick, just nude liner and a little gloss, but Laura learned to deal! It's hard to explain what Laura does exactly because she often does something counterintuitive to what I think I want. But she's so talented and dedicated that you trust her, and her magic takes over. It's unbelievable how much she has helped me understand my face.

Laura and I have been everywhere together—every hotel, every city, you name it. We're usually part of a trio rounded out by Serge Normant, the hair stylist and our dear friend. We enjoy each other's company, we love art and culture, and we're very much creatures of habit. None of us—Serge, Laura, or myself—like to go out. We do our work, head back to the hotel, order room service, and watch TV. What's bad about having professionals do your hair and makeup is that you forget how to do it yourself. On New Year's Eve, I tried to do my own hair and makeup and it was hilarious! I'm Laura-dependent! When I'm not working, I don't use much makeup, and I don't carry much with me. All I wear is mascara, Laura's camouflage product, and her gloss. I've gone to movie premieres, and that's all I have had on my face. I never, ever, ever leave the house without her camouflage. Never in my life. Since I've known Laura, I haven't done a film without it.

You know what else is amazing about Laura Mercier? She's worked incredibly hard to get where she is, but she hasn't succeeded on hard work alone. She utterly, utterly loves what she does. And I look all the better because of it!

—Sarah Jessica Parker

Sarah Jessica Parker by Michael Thompson

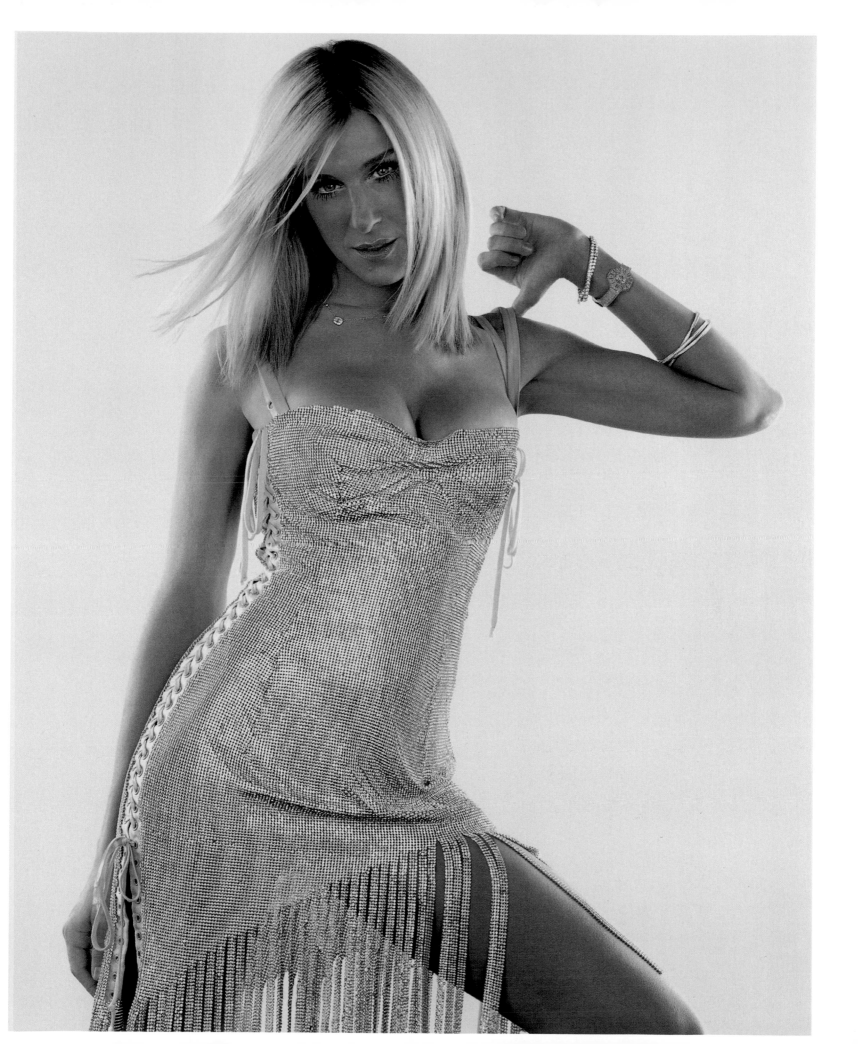

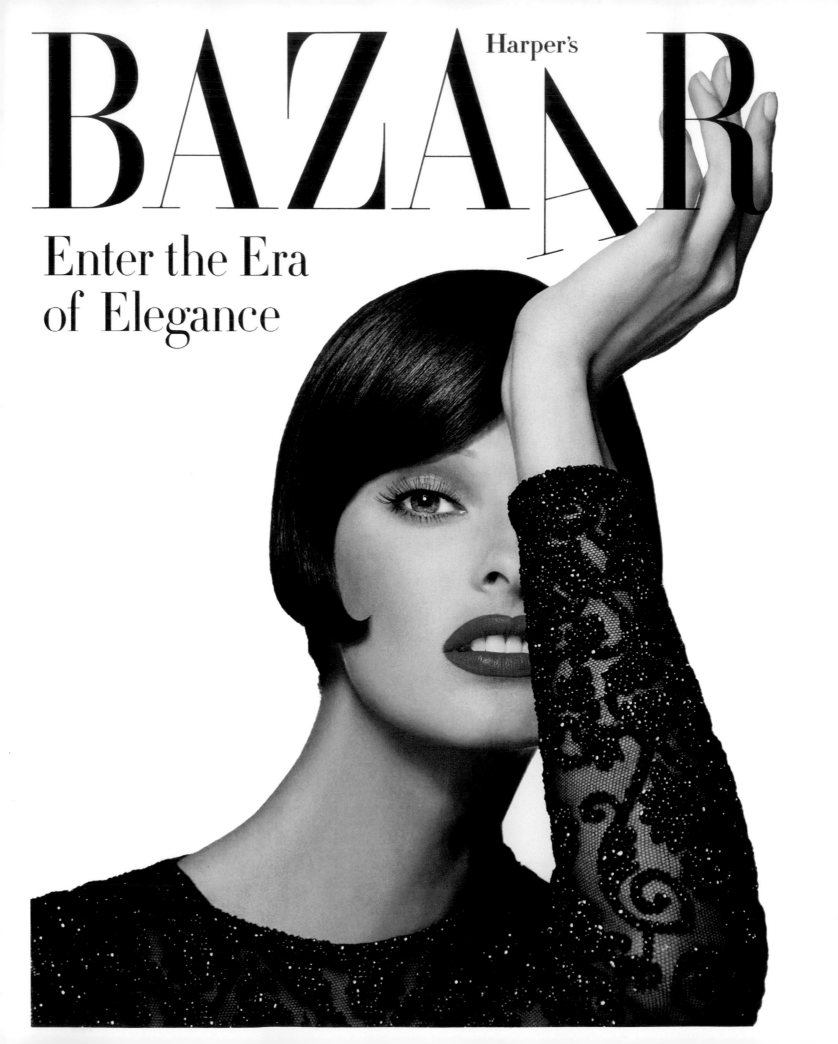

BAZAAR

Harper's

Enter the Era of Elegance

the new beauty secrets

Linda Evangelista by Patrick Demarchelier

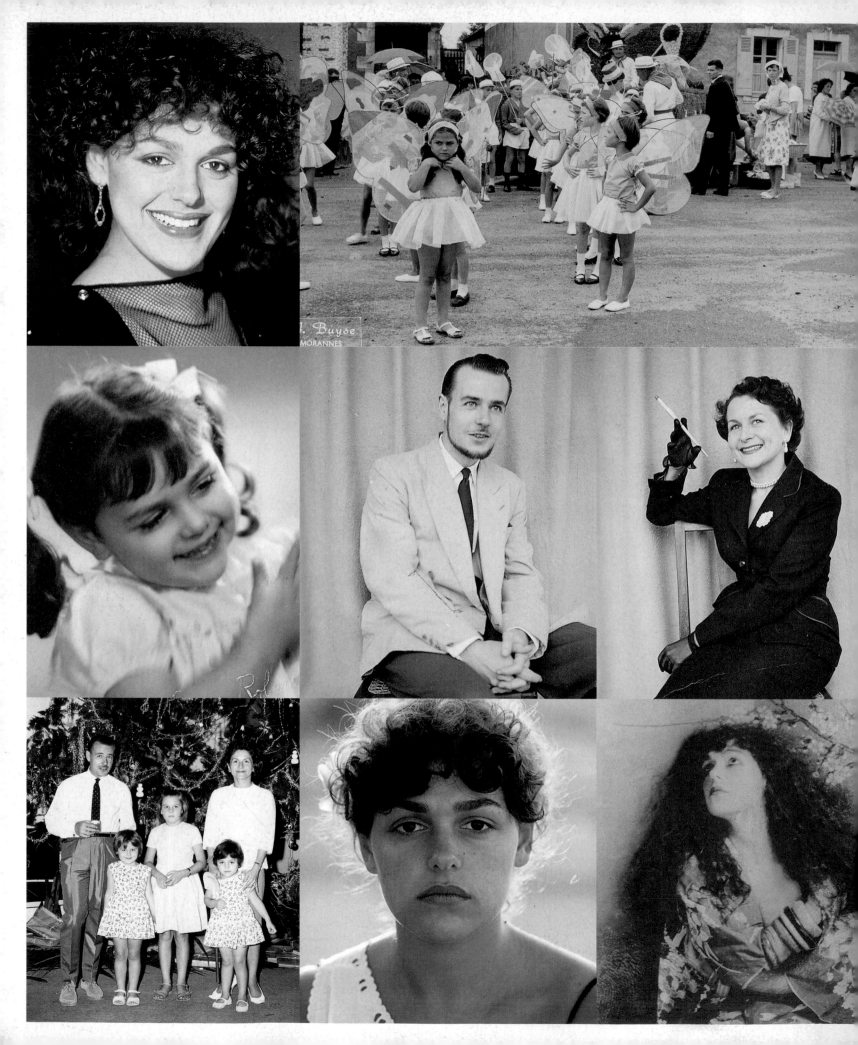

chapter one a life in beauty

I've been in love with beauty all my life, but I didn't set out to become a makeup artist. People are often curious to know how it happened, and the truth is that fate intervened. Many of my makeup artist colleagues dreamed of seeing their work in the pages of *Vogue* and *Harper's Bazaar* and fantasized about creating a signature line of beauty products, but I didn't. It takes confidence to envision that sort of future for oneself, and I just didn't have it. But what I did have was a little talent, a good work ethic, and the luck to have great mentors.

Since you've picked up this book, and *merci beaucoup* for doing so, I'd be honored for you to consider me *your* beauty mentor. Perhaps you're looking for tips and tricks so your makeup is the best it can be. If so, I think you've come to the right place. Since I got my start in the days before retouching pictures became so simple, I had to learn how to do makeup that was flawless. Once the pictures were printed, that was it, which is how my *Flawless Face* techniques (which I share in this book) and beauty products were born. I have perfected the techniques on everyone with whom I've worked and myself, for more than twenty years.

Perhaps you've picked up *The New Beauty Secrets* to update your look. I've had the good fortune to work with some of the most talented actresses, singers, models, photographers, hairstylists, and fashion editors and the photos we collaborated on have a truly inspirational quality that will motivate you to shake up your makeup routine. Whether it's Madonna's beautifully simple geisha face or Sarah Jessica Parker looking radiant and glowing in the ads for her signature fragrance, each picture has something timeless for you to take away.

Previous spread: Laura Mercier and her family.
Opposite: Laura and her beloved Jack Russell, Billy, as drawn by Izak.

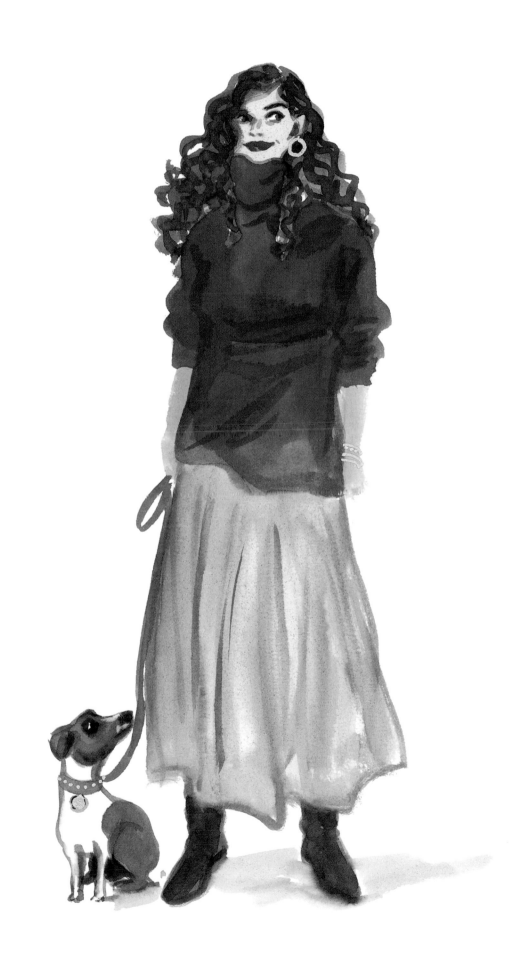

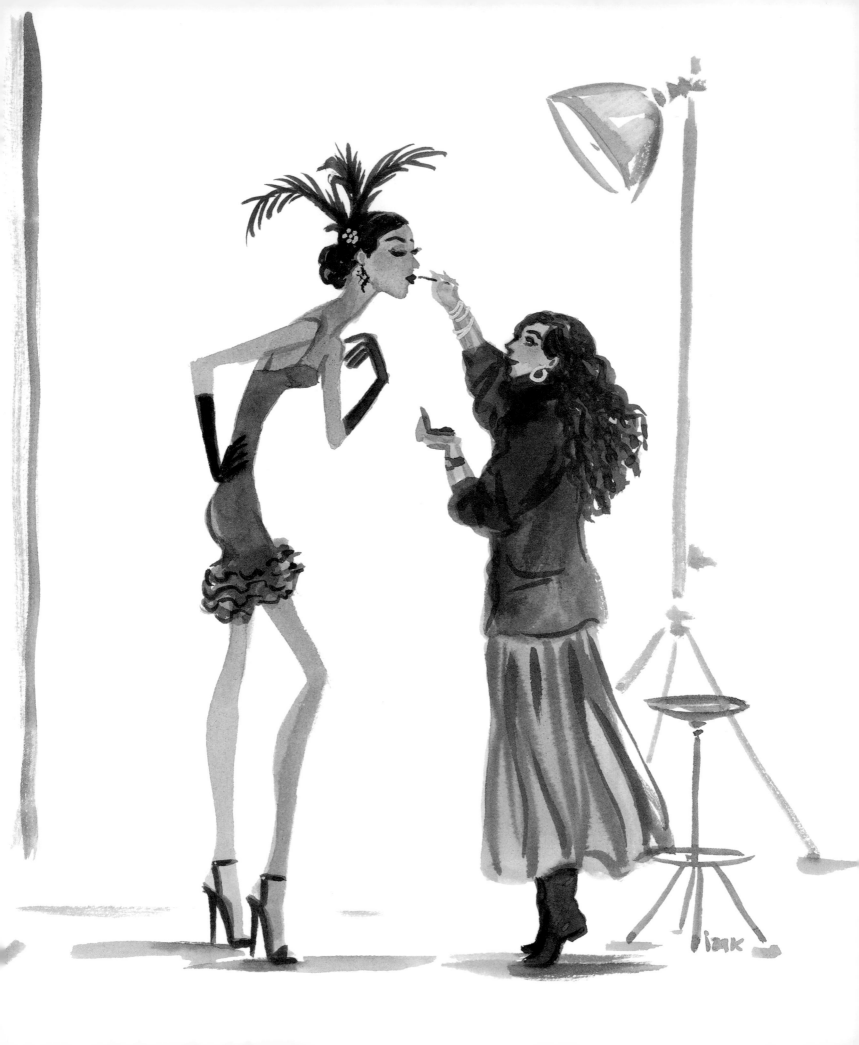

For me, beauty has never been about trends or making someone look weird just to be different. Aside from fantasy looks I created for music videos and certain magazine editorials, I was not the artist you hired to make models look freaky, nor are my makeup counters the ones you visit for blue lipstick or fuchsia eyeshadow. I've always been more interested in making women look as beautiful as possible while making them look like themselves. It always meant a lot to me to help others look their best, and because of this, I'd like to give you more than tips and pretty pictures. I want to help you find the key to being yourself and believing in yourself. It took me a long time to feel secure, and I'd like to share what I've learned along the way.

My story begins in Provence, the region of France that has inspired painters, perfumers, and so many others with its beauty. I was born Michèle Mercier (yes, my real name's not Laura!), the youngest of three daughters. As a child, I was a solitary creature drawn to all things creative. My passion was to draw and paint, especially faces. It allowed me to escape my reality. I had been diagnosed with severe asthma, and the high dosage of cortisone prescribed long-term for my condition caused a weight problem I struggled with for years. In addition, my grandmother had the "marvelous" idea to repeat constantly that I was so fat and ugly I would never get married! Now I can laugh about it, but at the time I did not.

Laura on assignment

Convinced of my shortcomings, I started to become obsessed by the beauty and charm of others. At the time, my mother and her friends were a constant source of fascination. Pretty and perfumed, they enjoyed entertaining in their homes, going to soirees, and dressing in the fashions du jour. Long before Linda Evangelista became a hair color chameleon, my beautiful mother went from brunette to redhead to blonde. She loved makeup, and I vividly remember her favorite green eyeliner on her green eyes and orange lipstick on her lips. When I was old enough, my mother let me apply her makeup for her. I loved the preparation and the ritual, but it didn't inspire me to focus on my own looks. If I could have put a potato sack over my head and worn that for the rest of my life, I would have been perfectly content!

I was planning to become a teacher of literature and language; but my creative side being so much stronger, I wound up attending art school in Paris. I had never been to the glittering city, but I moved there at the age of seventeen and lived in a tiny apartment I shared with a family of cockroaches. I loved school, and I loved living alone! Reality struck upon graduation when I realized I had no career path beyond starving artist. My mother suggested beauty school, of course, since I was so good at doing her makeup. It was probably the last thing I would have considered, but to her it was a perfect feminine profession.

I worried that my classes would be filled with girls killing time until they found husbands. Deep inside, I probably had the pretension of thinking of myself as an intellectual. Fortunately, my parents offered to pay for me to attend the Carita Institute, which was both a salon and the crème de la crème of beauty schools.

Laura and Billy on the go

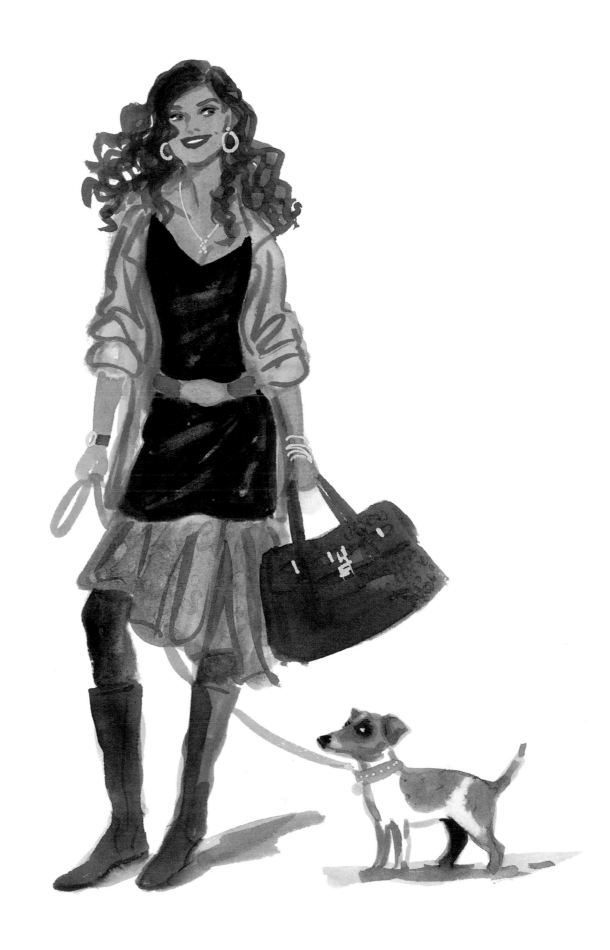

Here, beauty was taken seriously, thanks to the legendary Carita sisters, Rosy and Marie. The salon's appointment books were filled with the names of the rich and famous, from Middle Eastern princesses to British heiresses to French legends like Catherine Deneuve. It was a glitzy, glamorous world, and I felt as out of place as a sumo wrestler. Slowly, however, my confidence started to build. I was at the top of my class and truly interested in the different aspects of the beauty world, from dermatology to the application of makeup. I found a mentor, my makeup teacher Thibault Vabre, who was also a famous French makeup artist. After graduation, my parents asked Thibault if I could assist him because I was too shy to ask myself. To my shock, he said yes. I worked for him for a year and a half, organizing his powder puffs just the right way, cleaning his makeup kit, sharpening his pencils with a knife (because that's how he did it), and absorbing everything there was to learn about true makeup artistry. I kept remembering the words of an old friend: "No matter what job you do in life, whether it's something you expected or not, strive to become the best you can be!"

Thibault wasn't interested in teaching, so I took over his makeup classes at Carita and happily taught for three years. At the same time, little by little, I started to get my own bookings with magazines. Even though I was much heavier than I am today, with hair cascading to my bottom and a closet filled with shapeless black clothes, my reputation grew because I was professional, I was a perfectionist, and I was passionate.

Carita had a stable of hairdressers and makeup artists who represented the legendary beauty brand on photo shoots and in magazines, so Thibault, who was part of this select group, asked Rosy Carita to hire me. Rosy, impeccable and imperious with her dark, shiny chignon and bright red lips, had a few requirements. I needed to cut my hair, lose twenty pounds, and change my name. (Michèle Mercier was the name of a renowned French actress who was also a longtime Carita client.) Rosy preferred names ending in "a" (as Carita does) so she christened me Jessica and then Aurelia before Thibault convinced her to try Laura.

And so Laura Mercier was born. As weird as changing your name seems, it allowed me to shed my past and start over. I still had a lot of work to do on my self-esteem, and as part of the fashion world—a pretty cruel place to be when you're not the fashion type—I knew it wouldn't be easy.

In 1985, I decided to move to the United States. Terrified, I packed my bags and made the leap. I loved the United States because it was very far away from my past. You weren't judged as harshly as you were back in France, which is probably the most judgmental country in the world. I went to Weight Watchers, and it took me a year to shed twenty pounds, but I kept it off. Needless to say, things were hard, from the language barrier to the obvious cultural differences, but I kept in mind that you learned the most from the hardest experiences.

Little by little, my career progressed. Luckily, I got to the point where magazines were booking me to work with well-known photographers, supermodels, and the occasional celebrity client. At the same time, I was afraid to work with celebrities on my own. Working on them as part of a team was fine. The prospect of working with them *by myself* for film premieres, award shows, parties, and so on was so daunting. At the beginning of my career, I had a terrible experience with a renowned celebrity in France, and I never wanted to work with a famous face again.

One day, Steven Meisel, the brilliant fashion photographer and a good friend, finally convinced me to work with Madonna. Imagine! The night before I did her makeup, I actually spent hours in my bedroom throwing up. The first day we worked together, Madonna must have felt my anxieties because she did everything she could to make me feel relaxed. She encouraged me to be creative.

For the eight years we worked together, she was respectful and inspiring, and her impact on my confidence was tremendous, thanks to her intelligence and her sense of humor. I have many people to thank for the beautiful pictures in this book, but they might not exist if Madonna hadn't trusted me on that very first day. To be honest, it was the most valuable gift of my career because it cured my fear and gave me the confidence I never had before. I was able to move on and work with so many amazing people over the years.

So when you look through these pages and see the pictures of famous faces, you'll understand that there's much more to them than meets the eye, as they say. From my early days at beauty school to the creation of my makeup line a decade ago, it's been a very long journey and many of you have traveled part of it with me. I've met thousands of you in stores across the country during special events and appearances. Some of us have cried together, some of you have learned new beauty tricks from me, and some of you have taught me a few tricks. In the ten years since I launched the Laura Mercier line, you've inspired me so much. Now I hope to inspire you in every chapter with the knowledge that your personality and individuality are what count the most. In these pages, you'll definitely find realistic advice and simple tips for looking and feeling your best. But this is not a beauty encyclopedia. I want you to see how makeup can be fun and easy, but I'd also like you to understand how beauty is so much deeper than lipstick and powder.

Billy looks back

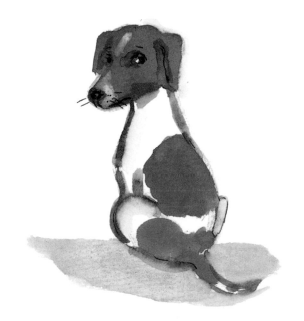

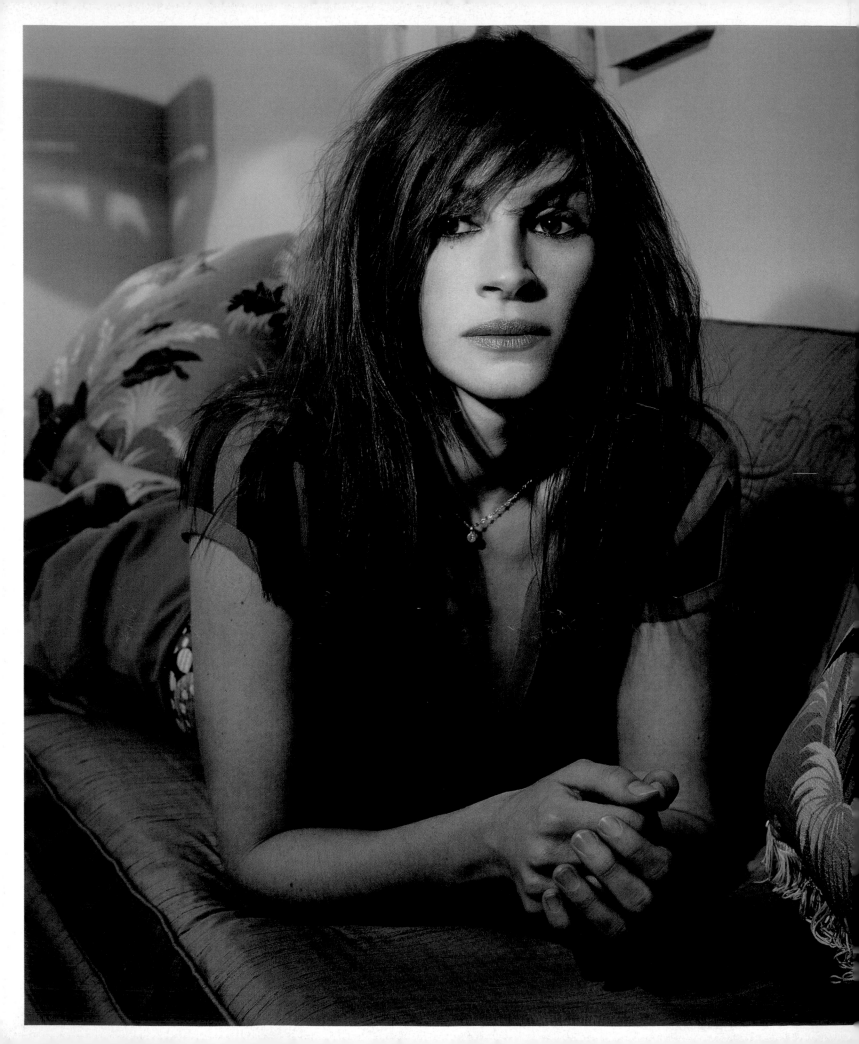

chapter two the new beauty rules

I'm not a big believer in rules. A few rules related to common sense things, yes. Many rules, no. As for beauty rules, I'm sure you've heard all the old ones. Don't wear red lipstick if you have red hair (one of my favorite looks!). Don't wear blue eyeshadow if you have blue eyes (not true!). Wear your blush a certain way if your face is a certain shape (very outdated!). When I was younger, beauty books advised you to hold a pencil against your nose to determine where you should tweeze your eyebrows. Have you ever tried that? It's been passed off as a universal rule, but we'd see many freaky eyebrows if everyone plucked according to those directions. It would be fine if everyone had the same face shape and the same eyebrows, but we don't.

The concept of beauty has changed so much throughout the past few decades that it's time for some new rules. The idea is to know what works for you and follow it. Look beyond the products and procedures that are popular and trendy; focus instead on what inspires you, enlightens you, and gives you confidence. Give *The New Beauty Secrets* a read, and see how they apply to your life. I hope you'll find a few things in this book that make you see yourself and the world a little differently.

1 What Makes You Unique Makes You Beautiful

Do you know how many people told Barbra Streisand to fix her nose? Or Cindy Crawford to have the mole on her face removed? Or Madonna and Lauren Hutton to fix the gap between their front teeth? Each of these amazing women was confident

Previous: Julia Roberts by Michael Thompson. Opposite: Christy Turlington by Michael Thompson. Such different faces, such modern beauties.

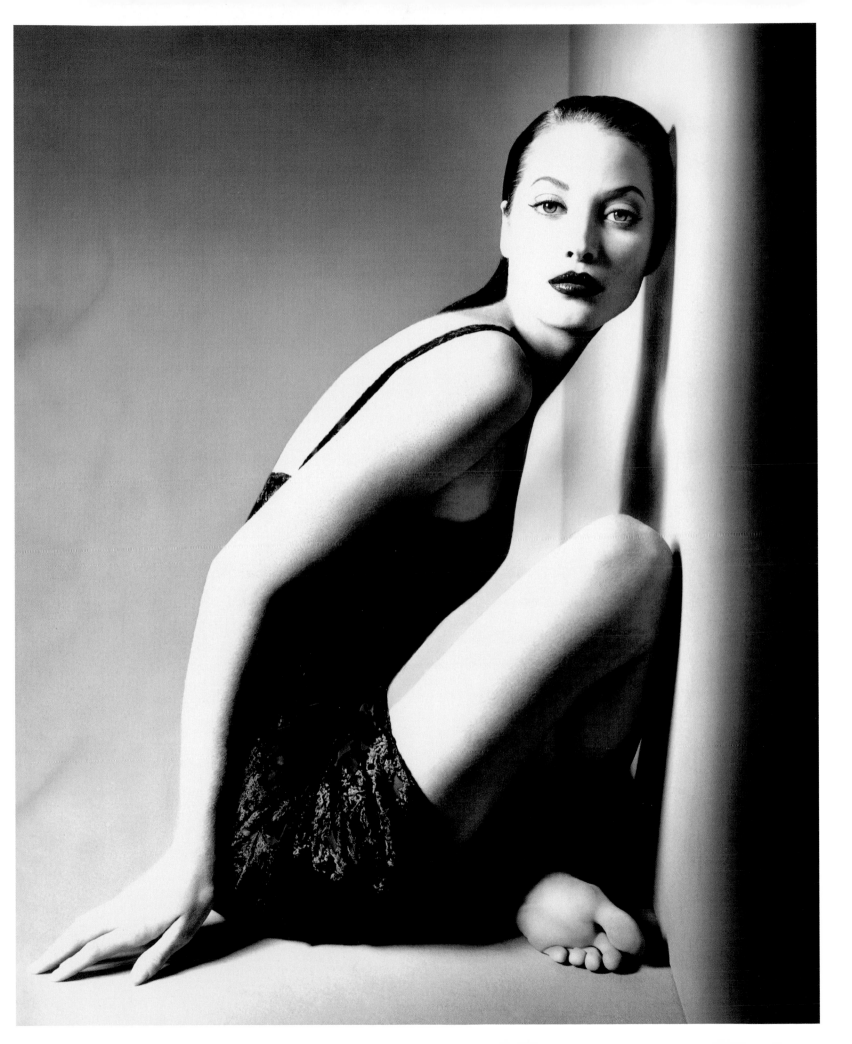

enough to refuse to change. They knew what so many women of true style understand: Beauty is not generic. *Quite often, the thing that makes you memorable is the thing that makes you different.* When you try to look and dress like everyone else, you merely look and dress like everyone else. Think of the women you admire. Do they blend in or stand out? If you were born a certain way, embrace it.

Change only what you can't live with, but try to accept who you are, and say yes to what makes you unique. Your confidence will make you sexier than any beauty product or accessory you could possibly buy.

2 Stop the Makeover Madness

We're trapped in a makeover-crazy world right now. TV programs, magazine articles, even books: Everywhere you turn, there's something about makeovers. Celebrities morph before our eyes, seeming to get blonder, thinner, and tanner overnight. I'm not crazy about the word *makeover* and the whole idea of "before" and "after." It always implies that there was something unacceptable with the "before." Although I think most everyone can benefit from a little concealer, blush, and lip gloss, my profession doesn't impair my objectivity. I believe some faces look just fine wearing nothing at all. A little makeup isn't the kind of change that hurts anyone. What I'm opposed to are the makeovers that favor a common look. They erase individuality and impose something that's not necessarily right for the subject and his or her lifestyle. Does everyone need the same stick-straight blonde hair? Does everyone need the same nose or the same size breasts?

That's something to think about if you're considering cosmetic surgery. So many of the women who come to my public appearances have questions and concerns about plastic surgery and want my advice. I'm reluctant to give it to them because I'm conflicted about plastic surgery. I know people who have benefited physically and mentally. They had a minimal amount of work done and felt great about the changes. I'm opposed to surgery that completely erases the original person. There are ways to tweak a nose, tighten a chin, and take some years off without making the person look like someone else. If you are interested in plastic surgery, you need to seek out the doctors who work hard to preserve individuality in a face.

Another thing that bothers me is the media's portrayal of plastic surgery as something easy and breezy when the reality is quite different. Makeover programs compress the recovery from months into minutes and imply that you'll return to your office in no time. It's not that simple at all. Despite the terms *plastic* and *cosmetic,* it's real surgery with all the implications and possible complications it entails.

Lastly, if you're thinking about plastic surgery, make sure you're getting it because *you* want to. Don't do it because you think you have to, and don't do it because your friends are doing it. Many women feel a sense of peer pressure today, and they don't want to be the "old" one among their acquaintances. Don't do it because you think your partner will find you sexier. Some women get surgery because they think it will save a marriage or a relationship, and that's rarely the solution. And definitely don't do it because you want to look like a celebrity. Do it if it's going to make *you* happier. If you think surgery is the answer to all of your problems, it's not.

I enjoy fashion magazines very much. It's fun to relax with your favorite ones, flip through the pages, and catch up on the latest fashions and trends. But you need to read them with a critical eye because they are as much about fantasy as reality. Yes, they are filled with factual articles that can help improve your health and your appearance and keep you up-to-date on events and personalities. At the same time, they're filled with pretty pictures that aren't always a true reflection of reality. Almost every picture you see in a magazine is retouched to some extent, whether it's an advertisement or part of the editorial.

You would be shocked if you knew what some photos look like in their original state. Computer retouching has made it possible to tweak every aspect of a picture. You can add or change the color of makeup; boost the color and texture of hair; perfect a complexion so it's porcelain smooth; whiten and straighten teeth; trim arms, legs, and torsos (instant lipo!), while making necks longer and breasts larger. Remember this information the next time you wonder why you don't look like a picture in a magazine.

Some celebrities such as Kate Winslet have spoken out about the extreme retouching practice (she was dismayed when a British men's magazine made her look thinner and taller for its cover), and some such as Jamie Lee Curtis have bravely pulled back the curtain to show the real "before" and "after" of untouched and retouched photos.

This isn't a reason to toss your magazines in the recycling pile and cancel your subscriptions. We all want a little fantasy from our magazines; otherwise, we'd just read newspapers and get the warts-and-all reality. I just want you to be aware so you're not comparing yourself with the people in the pictures. They may look beautiful and perfect, but it's a beauty and perfection that even the subjects of the pictures cannot attain. These photos are meant to entertain; they're not meant to be taken literally.

4 Be Smart About Celebrity

I said earlier that we're living in a makeover-crazy world, but that's nothing compared with the celebrity craziness going on these days. Magazines and TV programs are obsessed with celebrities: their shopping habits, dating, and every move. In turn, we've become obsessed! Is that a bad thing? That depends. It's ok to be inspired by some aspect of a celebrity's life, but do you know more about Angelina Jolie than you do about your own relatives? What's most damaging is when you start judging your own life and appearance against that of certain celebrities. Many women have told me they wish they had a body like this celebrity or had skin like that celebrity and so on.

Remember, under the designer clothes and the professionally applied makeup and styled hair, these are real women with the same insecurities as everyone else. In fact, many celebrities have said their public personas are "characters" they play and who have little to do with whom they really are privately. Just as we've discussed how plastic surgery won't necessarily improve your life and make your problems go away, neither will fame and fortune.

What helps is tapping into your inner celebrity. Think for a minute about what makes you fabulous and how you can celebrate it. Think about your appearance throughout the day. Do you spend a lot of time in sweatpants and old T-shirts? I'm sure you feel comfortable, but you could wear something from time to time that makes you feel more pulled together. Caring about yourself and your image can be more beneficial than you think.

5 Be on Trend Alert

Trends can be fun and inspiring, but don't let them dictate your style. If you love the pointy-toe shoes you bought last year and suddenly round-toe shoes are in, who cares? Keep wearing them. If a certain designer is hot, that doesn't mean you should wear his or her designs from head to toe. There's a term for that, and you don't want it to apply to you: *Fashion Victim.*

The Laura Mercier brand has always promoted substance and style in women, something to which you probably aspire since you are reading this book. We've never pushed trendy looks or products at our counters. There's a way to use trends appropriately, and it's not to let them use you! Have fun and use them as a way to change up your beauty or fashion routine. If you're stuck in a rut, there's no better way out than by incorporating something that's hot or of the moment, say an accessory or a color. With makeup, you run the risk of looking too extreme if you interpret a trend literally. Let's say bright purple eyeshadow is in and magazines show it worn across the entire eyelid. If you're intrigued, you can interpret the look however you like. You can try a sheer wash of purple shadow on your lids, line your eyes with purple eyeliner, or try some plum mascara on your lashes. You'll still be trendy, if that's important to you. At the same time, if a magazine declares something you love as out, over, or *so* last season, don't despair. Whether it's UGG boots, red lipstick, or your favorite pashmina from a decade ago, if it works for you, keep working it with confidence!

6 Sharpen Your Counter Intelligence

The beauty counter can be a great place if you approach it the right way. You can get free samples, try new products, ask for advice, and linger for as long as you like, playing with powders and lipsticks and perfumes. Chances are, you tend to avoid browsing the beauty counters unless you're looking for something new or specific. I don't blame you. The heavy-handed sales tactics and beauty associates eager to give you a spritz of a new scent or a makeover used to send me scurrying away as well.

We've tried to change that culture at Laura Mercier and make the counter experience more of a pleasant one, where women feel empowered and not preyed upon. When it comes to navigating the counters in general, here are a few tips to keep in mind. If you're just browsing, let the sales associate know in gentle but firm language. She probably works on commission, so you don't want to waste her time if you are not planning on buying anything. Not sure what you're in the mood for? Tell her you'll come find her if you need help. If you're looking for one specific thing, be clear about that. Know that the sales associate will suggest other products, either because they work in conjunction with the product you are buying, they seem like good products for you, or they're new. This doesn't mean you have to buy them! If you're not interested, you don't have to be aggressive or angry, which I've seen happen. Just say no thank you. And don't buy something because you're intimidated. You'll be reminded of how you felt every time you see the product in your bathroom cabinet or makeup bag.

We've all had the experience where we go shopping because we're depressed and we want instant gratification. We crave that comfort and reassurance so we head to the stores looking for a miracle and spend way too much money. I've been there many times myself. While I sometimes regretted what I spent, it made me feel good at the time. As long as this doesn't happen to you too frequently, it's ok!

7 Stop Apologizing for Your Appearance

Do you know how many women apologize when they meet me? They say "I'm sorry" as fast as they can to preempt any judgment I may make. They think I'm going to form an instant opinion based on their lipstick application, choice of eyeliner, and skill with a blush brush. Or worse, they apologize for things that are part of the natural aging process. Perhaps they're only doing this because they're slightly intimidated that I'm a makeup artist. It saddens me to think it's something they do with others as well.

Women need to be much kinder and forgiving to themselves and banish certain words from their vocabularies, such as droopy and ugly. Look in the mirror and notice the positive aspects of your appearance *before* the negative. I don't say this lightly because I know personally how difficult it can be for some women. It's impossible to change overnight, but once you get some positive ideas in your head, it will serve as an enormous factor for promoting yourself confidently in life.

If you define yourself by your looks, others will as well. Attractiveness shouldn't rate more highly than personality, talent, kindness, or intellect. Think about how you would like to be perceived and project that image, but be accepting of yourself. The wise words of Dr. Peter Reznik, a psychotherapist and a great friend who practices what he calls "mind-body integrative therapy" and who has helped me so much during my journey, come to my mind: "It seems that the further we go in the search of gaining more esteem, of having more than, being better than, being different from, the more alienated and unfulfilled we become." (Check out his great web site at www.drpeterreznik.com.)

Life's too short to let yourself get caught up in fashion, trends, plastic surgery, celebrity, or negative thoughts about yourself. It's fine to want to improve your appearance or your life and look your best, but don't use other people as the benchmark. Don't compare yourself with them and put yourself down in the process. If you take anything away from this chapter, it's that you need to be positive about yourself. If you already are, I hope you continue to have good self-esteem. If not, start small. Look in the mirror and focus on one good thing about yourself. Catch yourself in the midst of a negative thought and spin that sentiment into something complimentary. It's impossible to change your mindset instantly, but these little gestures will add up.

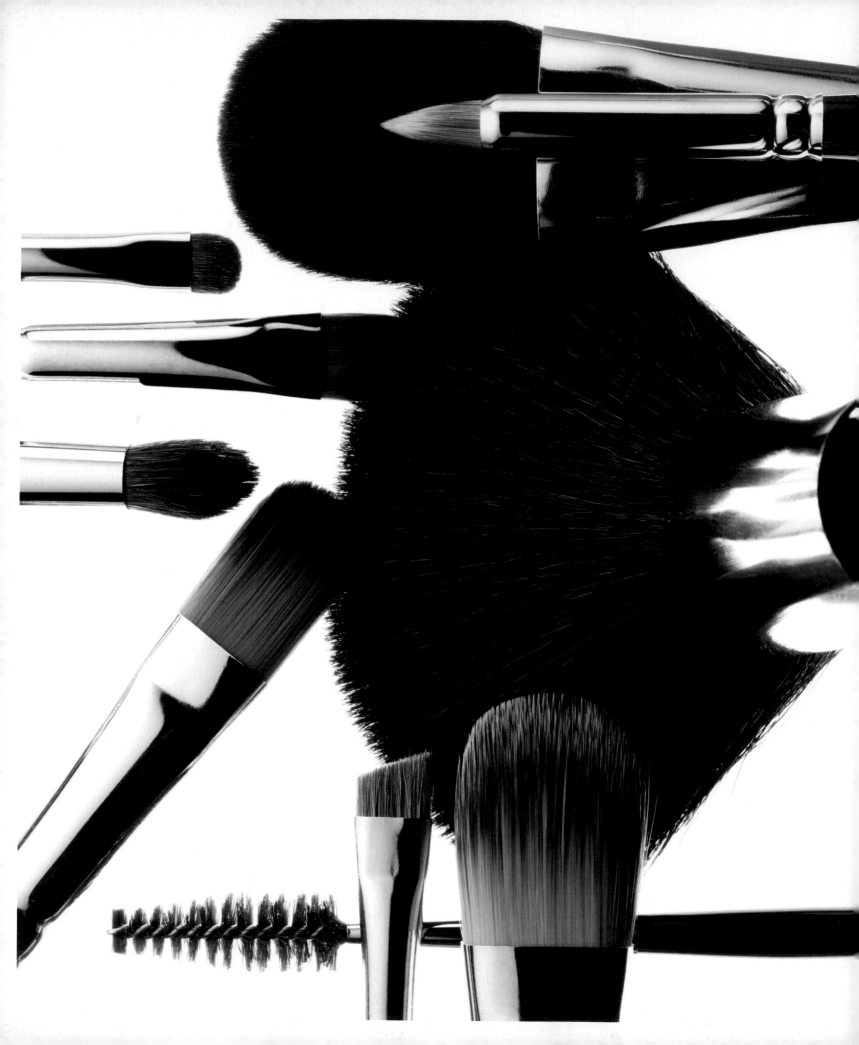

chapter three brushes and beauty tools

In the chapters ahead, I'm going to talk about a variety of beauty tools that you need to apply your makeup. These include brushes, foundation sponges, and velour powder puffs. Tools are available at a variety of price points, but the best ones tend to be on the expensive side. If price is an issue, buy only what you need. The tips and tricks in this book don't call for dozens of different brushes, and you can certainly make some brushes do double duty. Do try to buy the best brushes you can afford. If you take care of them, and I'm going to explain how, they can last for years. The oldest brushes in my makeup kit are more than twenty-five years old!

Washing Your Brushes

Caring for your brushes means washing them on a regular basis, not using them for a year and then tossing them. If you wait until your brushes look dirty, you've waited far too long. Apply makeup with clean tools; It's better for your brushes *and* your skin.

Basically, there are two kinds of brushes: those you use with creamy products and those you use with powdery products.

Let's talk about the first group, which includes brushes for concealer, camouflage, eyeliner, lip products, cream eyeshadow, and cream blush. These should be washed daily. This is a must for anything that touches your eyes or that you use to

beauty secret > Try applying your lip color with a brush. It gives you more precision when you contour or correct. It also results in a lighter coat than when you apply lipstick directly to your lips.

Linda Evangelista by Patrick Demarchelier

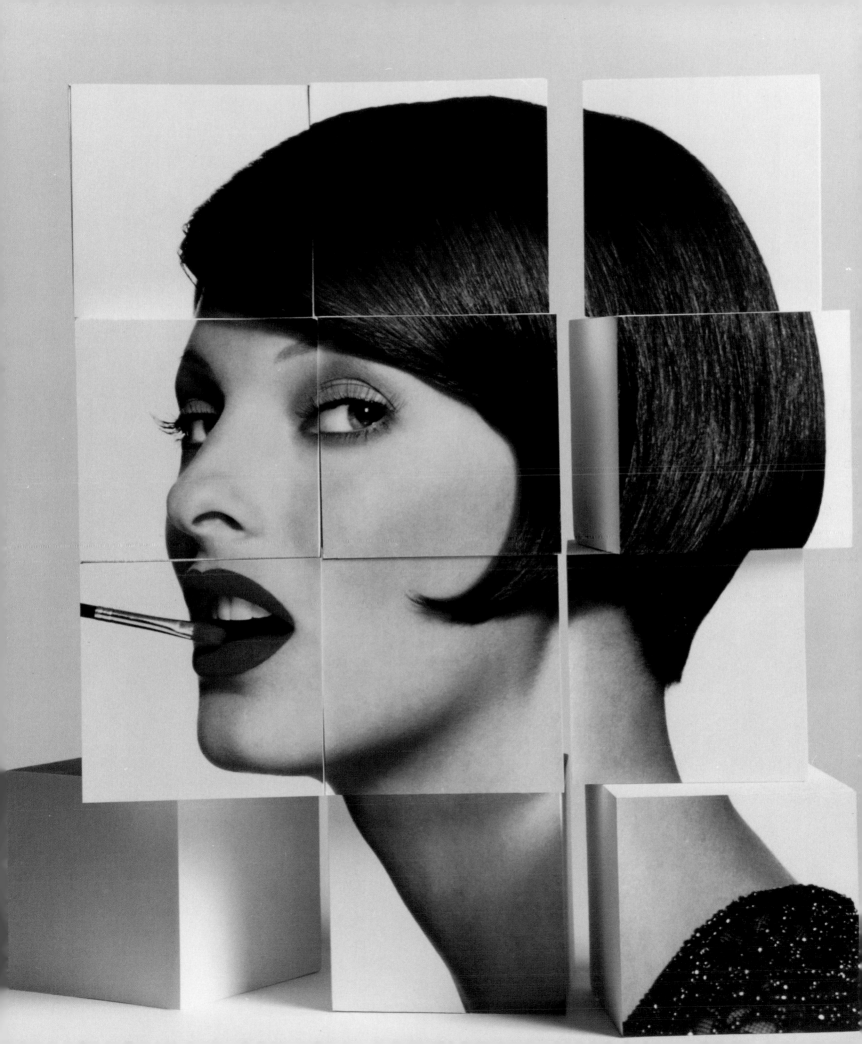

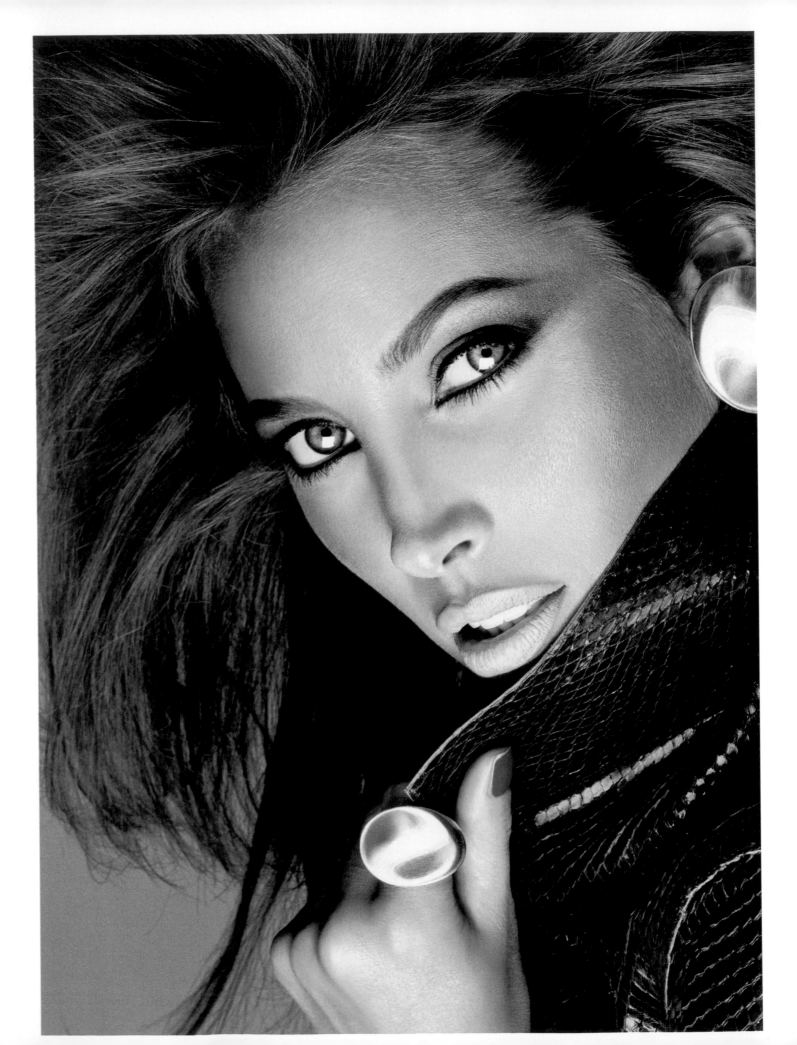

cover pimples because of bacteria. This probably sounds like a pain in the neck because you're so busy, and the last thing you need is another chore. But once you get in the habit, quickly washing the brushes will become second nature. You can wait until you come home from work to clean them, instead of doing it right after you apply your makeup in the morning.

beauty secret > If you have acne-prone or oily skin, wash your tools as often as possible. Your camouflage brush, for example, must be cleaned after every makeup application.

To get started you need some tissues and antibacterial dishwashing detergent. The detergent is perfect because it will disintegrate any grease or oil. Squeeze a little detergent on the brush and gently work it through with your fingers. Put the brush under warm running water and continue to work the soap through all the bristles in the direction of the hair, taking care not to bend the bristles. The soap will be creamy and opaque at first, then less so until you just have clear running water going through the bristles.

Put the freshly washed brushes on a paper towel or dish towel to dry, and reshape the brushes if necessary. For example, if a brush ends in a point, smooth the bristles back into a point. You can place the brushes near a heat source, like a radiator, but never directly on top.

For powder brushes, the directions are almost identical, with the exception that you don't have to wash them as frequently and you should use mild soap or shampoo. Again, be gentle. It's like washing your favorite La Perla bra, not scrubbing stains out of your jeans.

Christy Turlington, looking fierce and fabulous, by Michael Thompson

Sponges and Puffs

You should wash your sponges with mild soap under warm running water after every application. You should wash puffs in the same manner every few days or each week. Some makeup artists throw their puffs into the washing machine, but I don't recommend it. Most laundry detergents aren't mild enough, and all the tumbling around can damage them.

Put your sponges and puffs on a paper towel or dish towel to let them air dry. You may need to reshape your puffs.

Carry with Care

Do you travel with your tools? Maybe you take them to work every day, or perhaps you're going on vacation and want to bring them along. Make sure to have a nice case or brush roll in which to carry them. Don't toss them into your makeup bag where they'll get beaten up and dirty. Another option is to buy a travel-size brush kit that comes with a special carrying case.

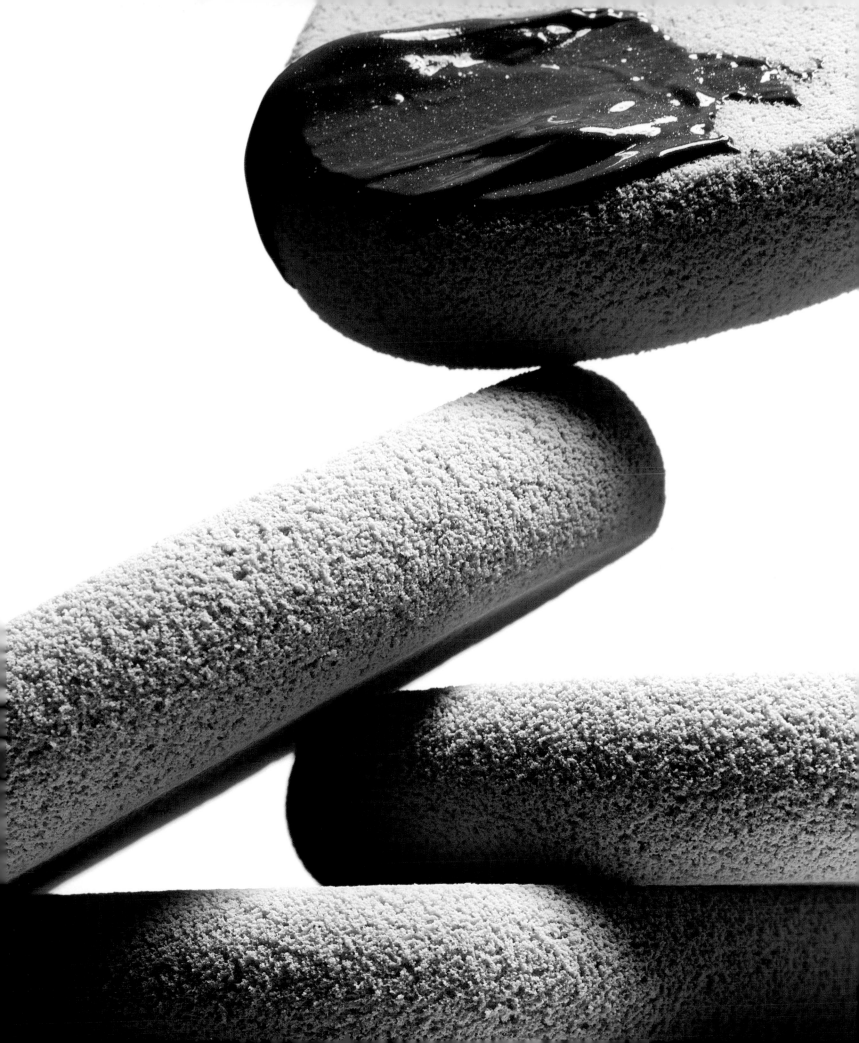

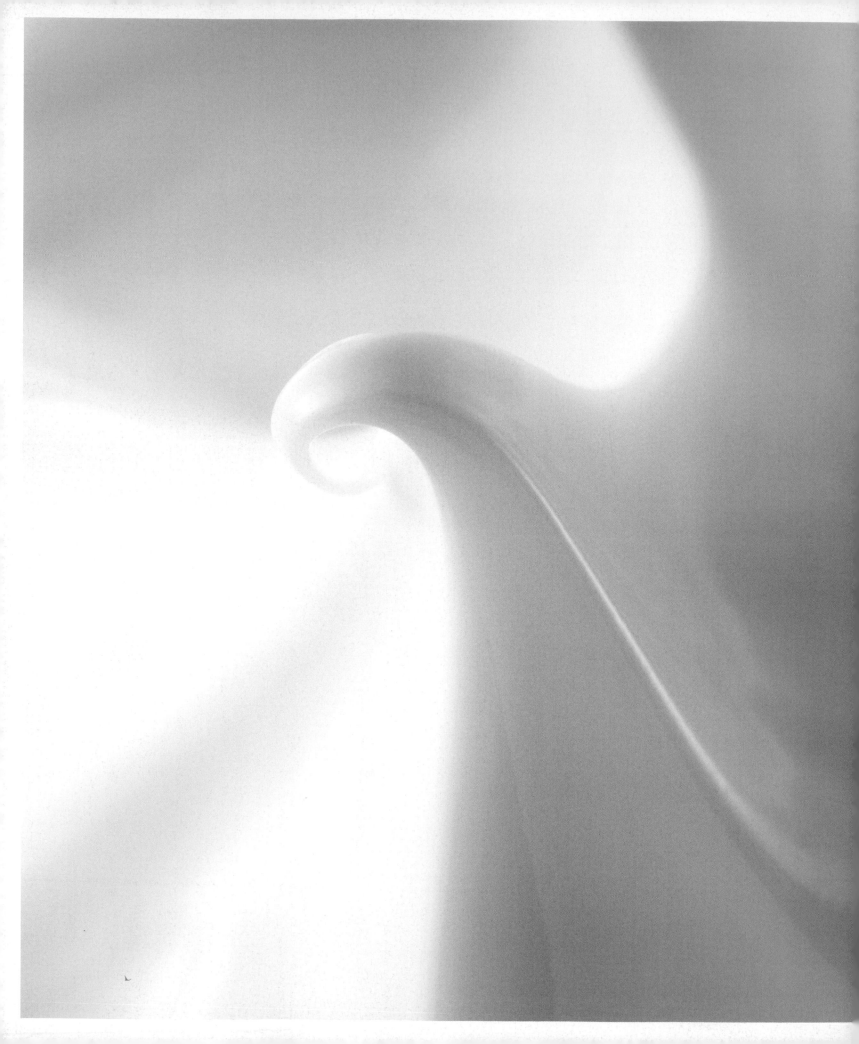

chapter four your guide to good skin

In the chapters ahead, I'm going to teach you how to get a beautiful complexion with makeup, so don't despair if you've got skin issues. And keep in mind that everyone, including me, has skin issues! Before I say a word about tricks and tips with cosmetics, we're going to focus on getting your skin in the best possible condition. It's easier to apply makeup to a face that is supple and prepared, like a canvas. If you slap powders and colors on a complexion that you haven't taken care of, it won't have the same effect.

When it comes to skincare, we're much luckier than the previous generation. There are better products on the market, drugs that can clear up acne, real wrinkle fighters, and better information about the effects of sun and diet. But how do you use those products and information? Are you smart about your skin? Lazy? Confused? Like so many women, you're probably a combination of all three. Whichever category you fit into, I've got information for you that I've gleaned throughout the years from the models and actresses with whom I've worked, from the dermatologists with whom I've consulted for my own skin problems, and from the scientists with whom I've worked to develop my skincare line.

Getting Started

Let's begin with some skincare 101. If you've already got a solid routine, you can read to brush up on the basics.

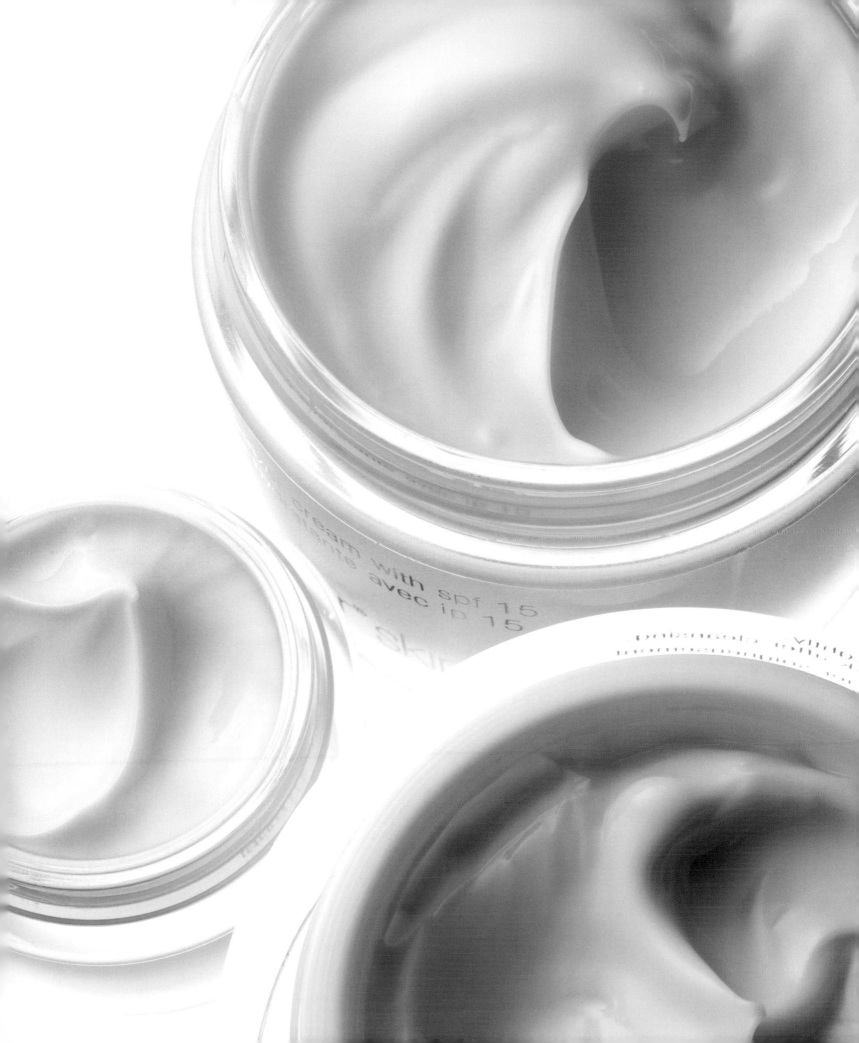

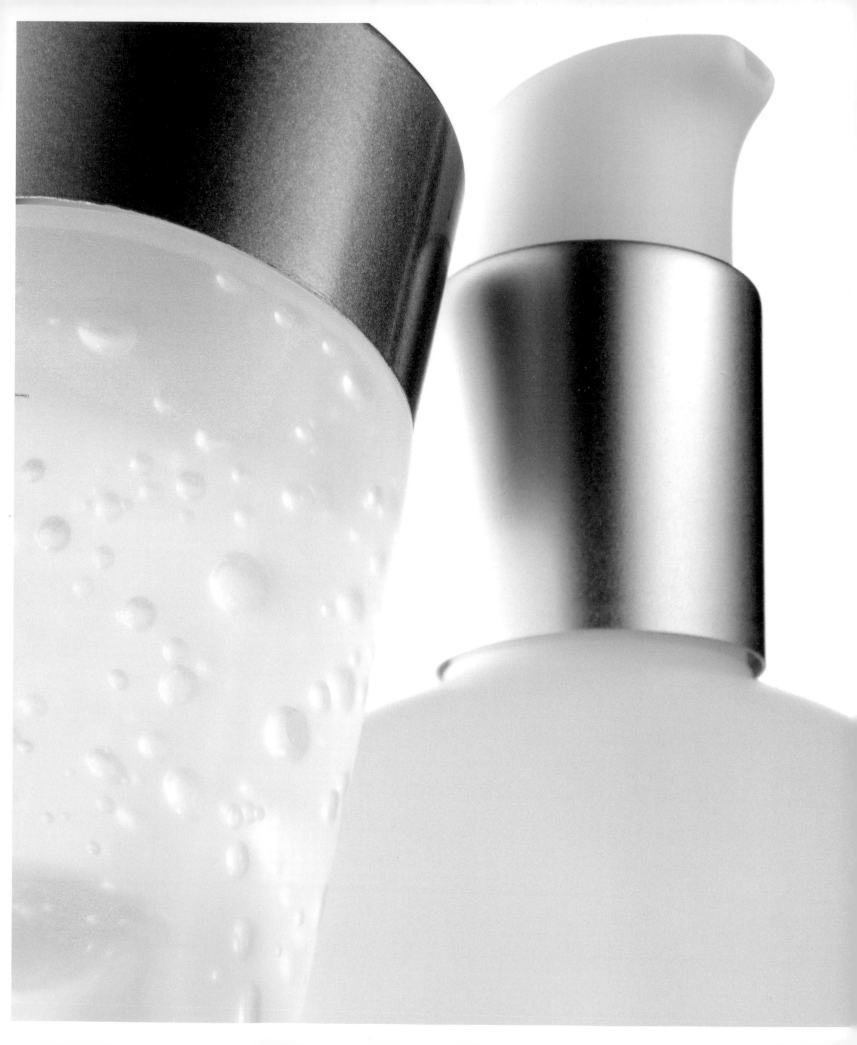

What You Really Need

A medicine cabinet filled with a dozen different jars, tubes, and bottles does not guarantee good skin. You can max out your credit card on the latest creams and serums, but the truth is you need only a few things. Maybe you love skincare and trying the newest items is a passion of yours. That's fine, but don't be a skincare shopaholic because you worry about missing the one item that will make all the difference in the world. It doesn't exist yet, and when it does, we'll all know, because Oprah will probably tell us.

Regardless of your age, your face can fare very well with a few targeted items, listed as follows:

Moisturizer with SPF for day

Moisturizer without SPF or a night cream for night

Eye cream (unless you're a teenager)

Serum or a solution-oriented layering product

Makeup remover

Cleanser

These are the basic products you should use on a regular basis. We'll talk about extras, such as masks, acne fighters, and exfoliators, later in the chapter.

Your A.M. Routine

1 If you've cleansed properly the night before, you don't need to wash your face when you wake up. Splashing your face with water is just fine, although I personally like using a light cleanser. It makes my skin more supple and opens the pores so they can absorb moisturizer.

2 Apply your serum or treatment product if directions specify daytime *and* nighttime usage.

3 Apply your moisturizer with SPF or you can use a separate sunscreen if you're going to be exposed to very strong sun. If you want to wear makeup over your sunscreen, make sure it's a lightweight sunscreen. Some sunscreens are not compatible with makeup, and it's difficult to apply products on top of them.

beauty secret > Consider changing your products seasonally, which is something I've always done. In the warmer months, a light lotion may be better for your skin than a heavy cream and you may want to use a higher SPF. If you're going to spend time outside, also consider using an SPF stick made especially for eyes and lips. If sunscreen tends to make your eyes sting, this will give you protection without the pain because it doesn't run or migrate as easily. In the colder months, with dry heat inside and frigid, damp conditions outside, a richer cream may be the way to go.

4 Apply your eye cream under your eye only. It's not necessary to use it on your eyelid in the morning, and it will interfere with any eye makeup you are wearing.

Jennifer Lopez, so fresh faced and sultry, by Michael Thompson

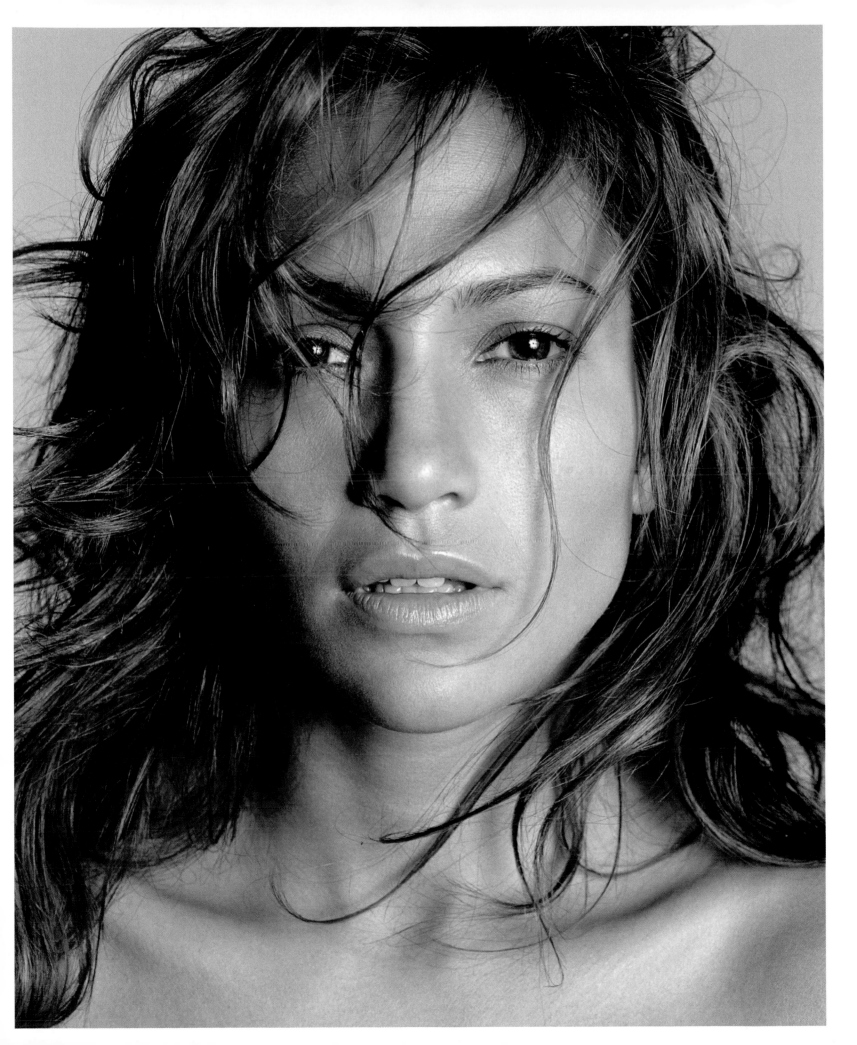

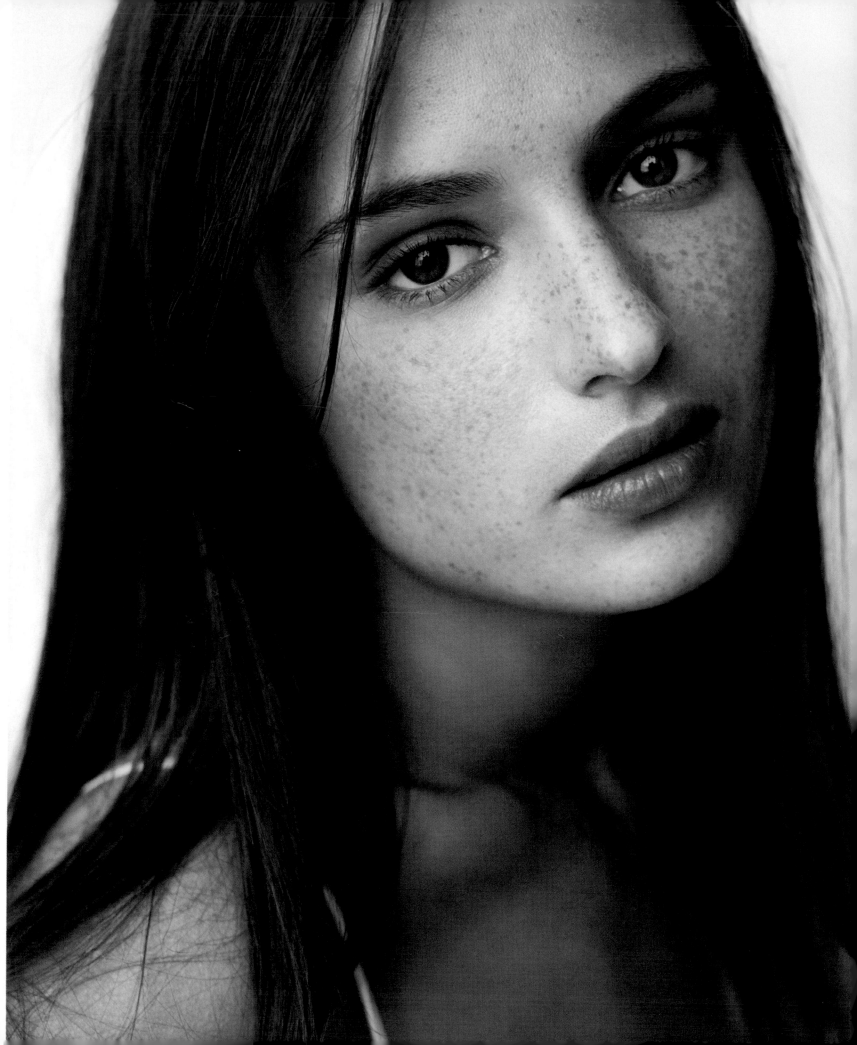

Your P.M. Routine

1 Before you go to bed, you *must* wash your face. Otherwise, you're asking for blackheads, breakouts, and flare-ups. Do you really want to fall asleep with all that accumulated dirt, pollution, bacteria, and makeup on your face? This is something I've always been very good about. During my wilder days, when I'd come home at six in the morning after dancing all night, I'd always wash my face. I couldn't stand the idea of my dirty face touching my pillow. If washing your face every night isn't a habit for you already, it will become one over time, just like brushing your teeth.

If you're not wearing much makeup, use a cleanser that doubles as a makeup remover. Make sure it's a cleanser for your skin type and one that doesn't contain too much fragrance and detergent. You don't need those things when you just want to clean your face. If you are wearing makeup, use a specific remover and some quality cotton pads to get everything off, especially your eye makeup. Follow with a cleanser for your skin type and pat your face dry.

2 If you're using a serum or special treatment product, then the time to use it is after cleansing. (If you prefer, you can skip this step and move right to moisturizing.) Generally, serums go under your moisturizer. Use a few drops or as much as directed and smooth onto your skin. Unless directions specify that you must use day and night, you can reserve this step for your P.M. routine and use once a day.

Freckles can be beautiful. Don't feel compelled to cover them. Photo by Patric Shaw.

3 Moisturize with a cream or lotion that's SPF-free (you certainly don't need SPF at night!) or a night cream. Don't slap the cream onto your face, neck, and chest; really massage it in. That doesn't mean using half the contents of the jar, but taking the time to literally push the amount of product you need for your skin type into your pores while they are still open and boost the circulation to your face in the process.

4 Apply your eye cream gently around your entire eye area, including your eyelid, but be careful not to get it into your eye. Again, take the time to really work it into your skin. Look for an eye cream that is packed with benefits, not one that simply moisturizes.

beauty secret > Not familiar with serums? This is a category of product that has become very popular throughout the past decade. Basically, serums are concentrated potions that contain antioxidants, vitamins, wrinkle fighters, firming agents, you name it. Some serve very specific purposes, such as collagen boosting, while more of them are multipurpose. Some women use them alone, but serums are generally designed to wear under your moisturizer. Do you need a serum? This is completely up to you. They can provide benefits that your moisturizer can't, and they certainly won't hurt. Find one that targets your specific skincare needs and start road testing it.

Heather Graham, looking luminous in a tiny bit of makeup, by Michael Thompson

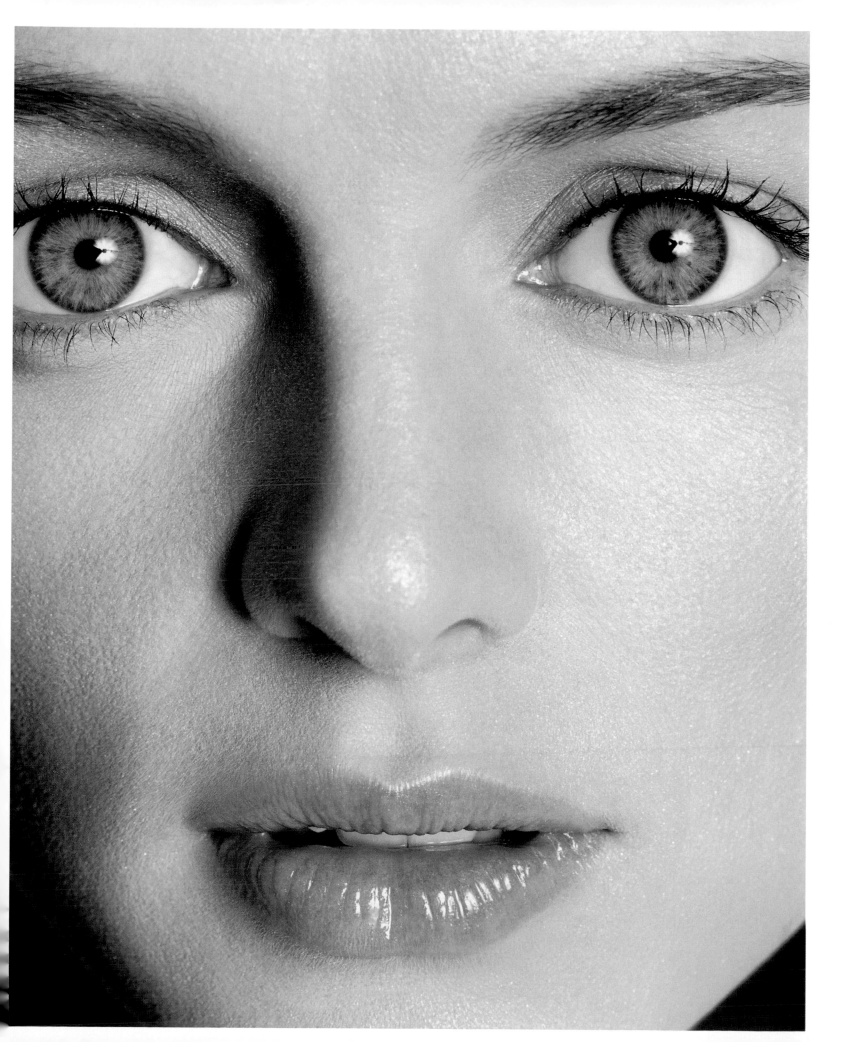

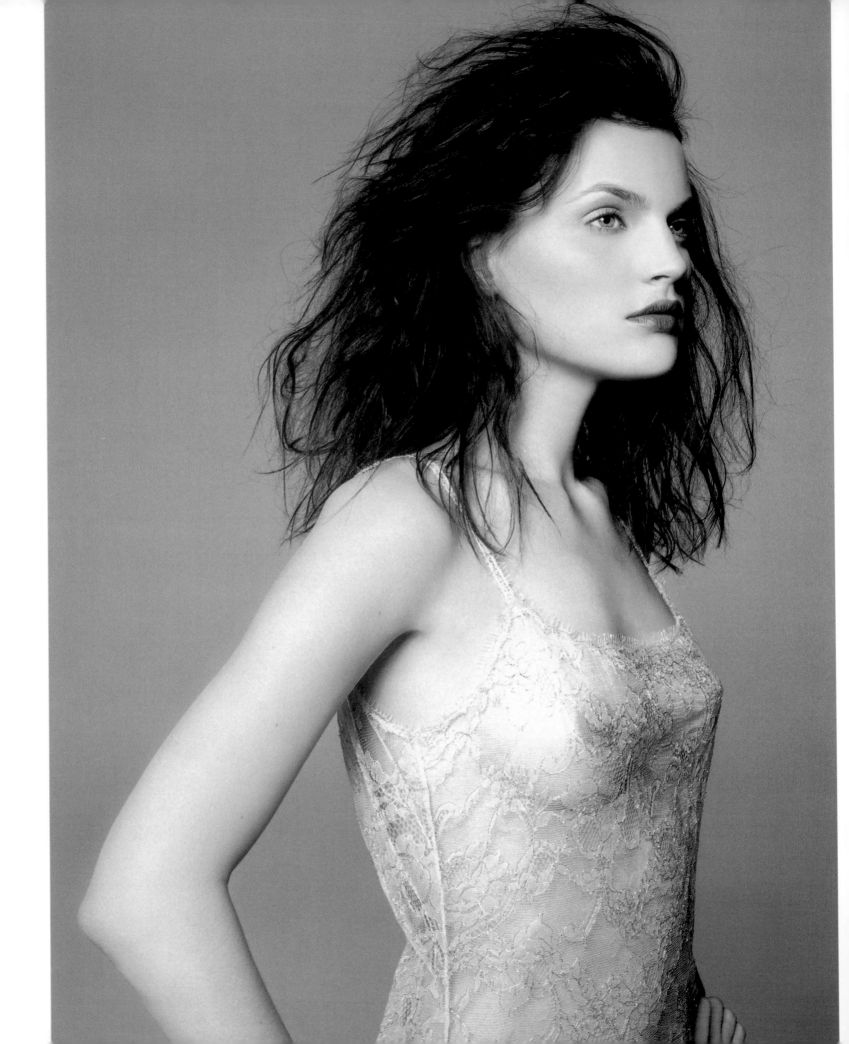

beauty secret > I remember a friend's grand-mère who was meticulous about facial massage. She had a yellowed newspaper article on facial massage from the fifties tacked to the wall in her bathroom, and she would follow the steps every day and night. I don't know if it worked, but she looked wonderful. Perhaps it was the massage or the fact that she took the time to really care for her face. My friend's grand-mère didn't realize it, but her approach was very Zen in that she completely focused on doing something perfectly. That concept appeals to me because I'm not a natural multitasker. I try to do my best in everything I do, but I do one thing at a time, whether it's making my tea in the morning, cleansing my face, or applying my makeup.

You can do a simple version of facial massage by remembering a few rules. When applying moisturizer to your face, use gentle upward strokes. When applying to your chin, throat, and chest, use downward strokes.

It's that easy. Just eight simple steps for day and night. Follow these meticulously, and you will be rewarded with a better complexion. Of course, this may not be enough if you have problematic skin, so we'll discuss additional steps you can take and go further into detail about smart skin practices.

Guinevere by Michael Thompson

It's possible that you're abusing your complexion and you don't even know it. Believe it or not, you could be taking *too much* care of your skin. What are the signs? Well, how many of the following things do you get or use on a regular basis?

Microdermabrasion

Glycolic washes

Chemical peels (at home, doctor's office, salon, or spa)

Retin-A or retinol products

Alpha hydroxy acids (AHA)

Exfoliant/Scrubs

Laser treatments

Your skin is going to break out, become increasingly sensitive, or both if you do too many of these treatments. I meet so many women who feel the items above are simply part of a modern skincare routine. They're left with raw, flaky skin that doesn't look good, and they don't understand why. If this is happening to you, answer this question: Does your skin look better now than it did before you tried any or all of these treatments? If so, fine. If not, it's time for a simpler routine. If it's a prescription skincare product that's the problem, stop using it and talk to your dermatologist. Perhaps you need a lower dosage, or you should use it sporadically. Many women are afraid to question their doctors' orders. Just because something is prescription only, doesn't mean it's better.

Jodie Foster by Steven Meisel

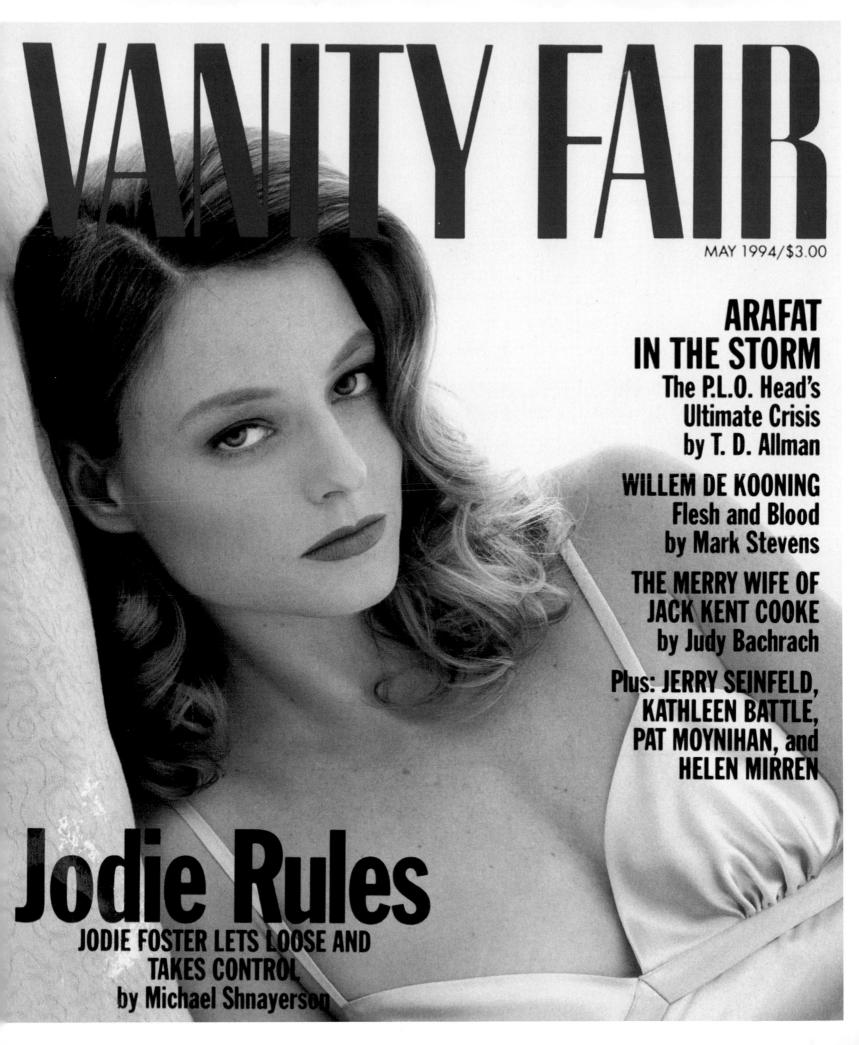

VANITY FAIR

MAY 1994/$3.00

**ARAFAT
IN THE STORM**
The P.L.O. Head's
Ultimate Crisis
by T. D. Allman

WILLEM DE KOONING
Flesh and Blood
by Mark Stevens

**THE MERRY WIFE OF
JACK KENT COOKE**
by Judy Bachrach

**Plus: JERRY SEINFELD,
KATHLEEN BATTLE,
PAT MOYNIHAN, and
HELEN MIRREN**

Jodie Rules

**JODIE FOSTER LETS LOOSE AND
TAKES CONTROL**
by Michael Shnayerson

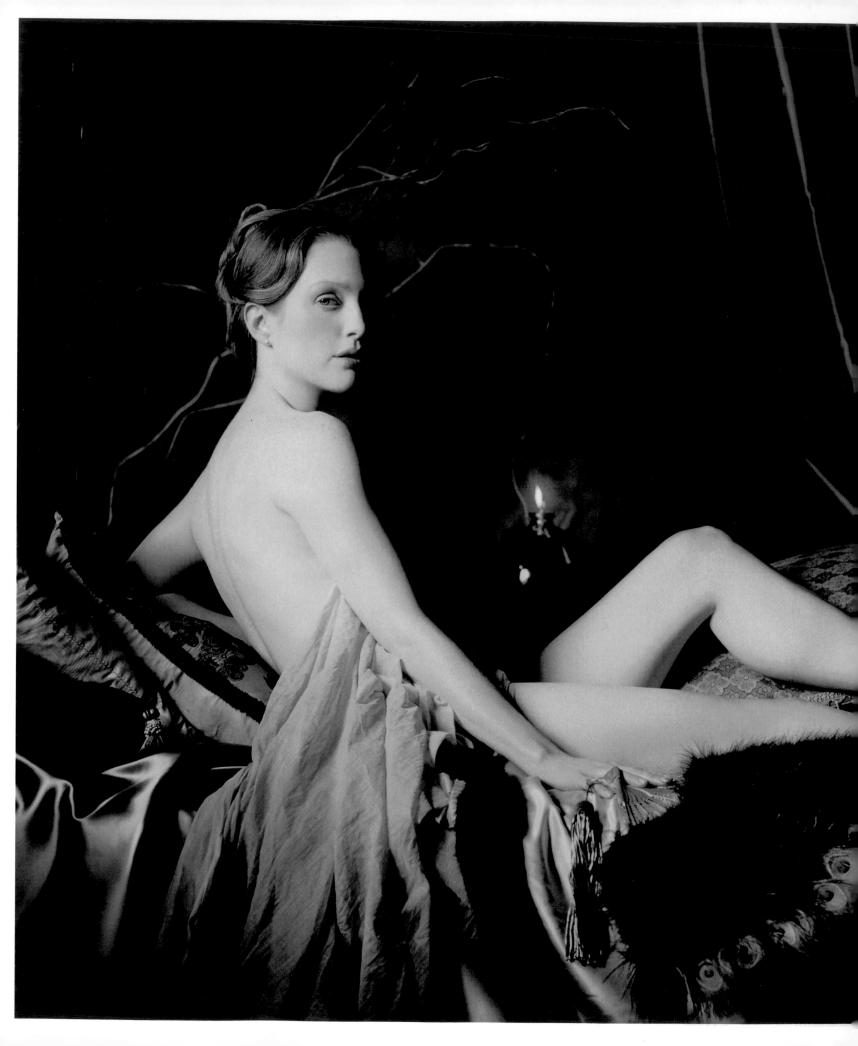

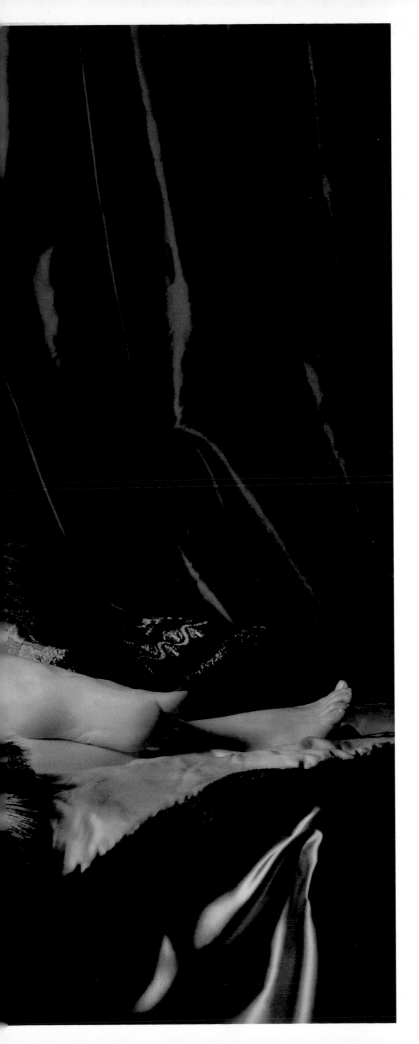

Laura makes women look the way they want

to look—healthy, smart, really pretty, and

strong. She never overdoes your features.

—Julianne Moore

Julianne Moore by Michael Thompson

The Truth About Expensive Skincare

Just because there's an astronomical price tag attached to a fancy jar of cream doesn't mean the pricey potion is superior to less expensive products. Personally, I thought it was crazy when companies started offering face creams for $500. Now brands are introducing exotic moisturizers and antiaging serums for $1,000 and more! Trust me when I tell you that this has more to do with marketing than the price of the ingredients. I've worked in skincare laboratories with researchers and scientists to develop products, and I haven't come across any ingredients yet that justify that kind of money. There is very good skincare available today for under $100.

Smart Skin Food

Instead of a $1,500 cream, let's talk about a $5 pint of blueberries or a $3 bag of spinach. Your diet is an important part of your skincare regimen because the health of your skin and the foods you eat are directly related. Much of this is common sense. Try to reduce the amount of fried and sugary foods that you consume. Make sure you get enough leafy green vegetables and brightly colored fruits and vegetables. Everyone's heard about the importance of omega-3 essential fatty acids, so make sure to get some salmon or other oily fish into your diet. Lastly, give your beverages some thought, and make sure you're drinking enough water and not too much soda.

I don't want you to be obsessed by food or diet. Nothing should be an obsession in life, but try to find some sense of balance for the sake of your skin.

Probably the best news about modern skincare is that you don't have to suffer from acne anymore. For the worst cases, there is Accutane, a very powerful drug that dries up your skin and clears acne in the process. (Take Accutane only under the supervision of a dermatologist; never use a friend's prescription or buy it online.) There's also Proactiv, a line of products specifically designed for acne-prone skin that has helped many people, including many celebrities. These are strong but effective options.

If you have acne, it can be maddening, especially if you're not a teenager anymore. Adult acne is becoming more and more prevalent. I suddenly developed adult acne at the age of twenty-six, even though I was taking excellent care of my skin. It drove me crazy, and I did all the things you're not supposed to—stress over it, pick at the breakouts, and so on. As a makeup artist, I spend a good part of my day fewer than six inches from someone's face. Being that close to people only made me more self-conscious about my complexion. Fortunately, the situation improved with the help of a dermatologist, but I learned how frustrating and debilitating a serious skin problem can be.

If you suffer from acne, then put together a plan of attack. Don't pick at your face, and don't strip it dry by overusing cleansers, astringents, and pimple creams. Consult with a dermatologist, and determine the routine and products that will work for you. If over-the-counter products are the only option, look for ingredients like salicylic acid, which helps prevent future breakouts. Benzoyl peroxide helps clear existing breakouts, but it can dry the skin so use it sparingly and according to the directions.

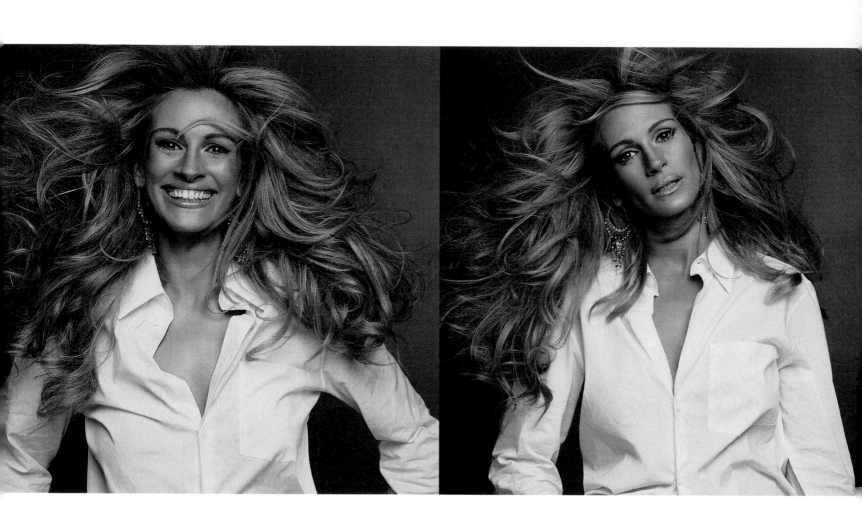

Julia Roberts by Laspata DeCaro

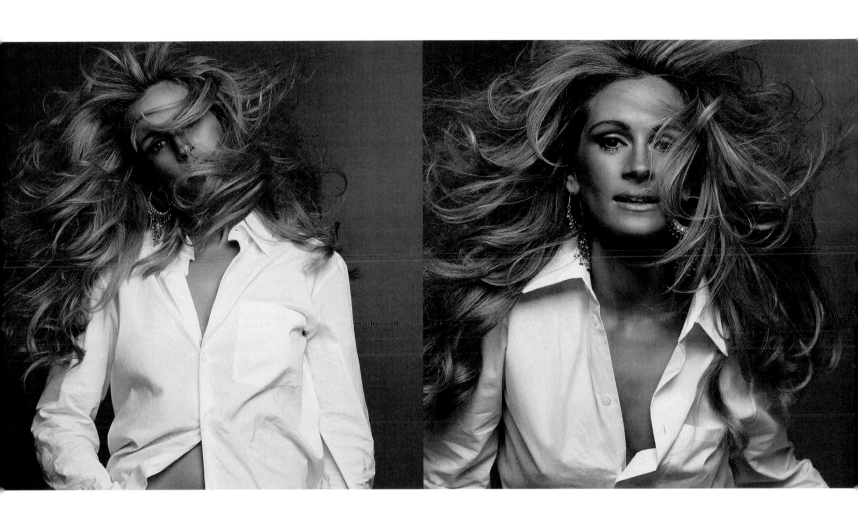

The following are a few common sense things you can do as well:

- Stick to a skincare routine like the one I described earlier.
- Keep your hands and your phone off your face during the day. Many women press their phones into their faces and don't realize it.
- Keep your hair off your face.
- Pay attention to your diet. Follow a healthy eating plan, but also monitor your diet to see if certain foods trigger your acne. Sugar and alcohol can be bad, as can some dairy products.
- Get enough sleep.
- Try to reduce your stress level. Most of today's adult acne is triggered by stress, so try different things to de-stress—massages, deep breathing, meditation (even five minutes a day!), yoga, listening to a soothing CD, or taking a long, hot bath.

The Rosacea Epidemic

Acne's not the only skincare problem on the rise among adult women. I see more women dealing with rosacea these days. According to www.rosacea.org, a very useful web site run by the National Rosacea Society, more than fourteen million Americans are affected. Rosacea is characterized by redness on the cheeks, nose, chin, and forehead plus bumps, pimples, and visible blood vessels on the face. It's an uncurable condition that is painful both physically and emotionally, but you can keep it under control. If you're affected by rosacea, there are certain oral and topical medications your doctor can prescribe, but you also need to be on the lookout for things that trigger your flare-ups (for example, alcohol, extreme weather conditions or temperature, and certain foods). In terms of beauty products, you should avoid harsh scrubs, anything irritating (Retin-A, Renova, retinol products, glycolic washes, and so on), and anything containing heavy fragrance. In Chapter 5, The Flawless Face, I'm going to give you some tips for covering your rosacea and dealing with the makeup issues particular to that condition.

Oily Skin

If you have oily skin, chances are you are scared of moisturizer. That was a legiti-mate fear back in the days when formulas were heavy, but today you have fabulous lightweight lotions. You actually do need moisturizer if you have oily skin. For some para-doxical reason, the oil on the surface of your complexion does not moisturize your skin.

Whatever you do, don't get too aggressive with your skin. It's very easy to strip your skin with foamy cleansers and medicinal toners. That tight, dry feeling might be a relief, but it's not going to solve the problem. Stripping the skin will only cause more oil production or could lead to our next issue: dehydrated skin.

Dehydrated Skin

This is another condition I'm seeing more of lately. It's not the same as dry skin. It's very easy to recognize because the skin feels like parchment or paper and can have some flakiness. Climate, travel, and stress exacerbate the problem, which comes from abusing the skin with chemical exfoliants and not moisturizing. Believe it or not, there are women who think buying moisturizer is like throwing money out the window. It's not because they're frugal and pinching pennies. These are women who shop in the best department stores and wear makeup on a regular basis; they just don't want to waste time putting on moisturizer, and their skin is prematurely aging as a result. If your skin has that dry, crepey feeling, then it's time to start moisturizing day and night.

Fun in the Sun

How do you protect your skin from the sun? Maybe you don't bake at the beach anymore, maybe you never did, but you still need SPF in your life. You get unintentional sun exposure all the time, whether you're shopping at the flea market or running errands outside. At a minimum, you should wear a moisturizer that contains SPF 15 on your face, neck, *and* chest. (Anything less than SPF 15 isn't worth it in my book.) So many women forget about their chests, and I see a lot of sun damage there. If your shoulders, arms, and legs are going to be exposed to the sun, you'll need sunscreen there as well, and you can never go wrong with a hand cream that has SPF in it.

Meg Ryan by Patrick Demarchelier

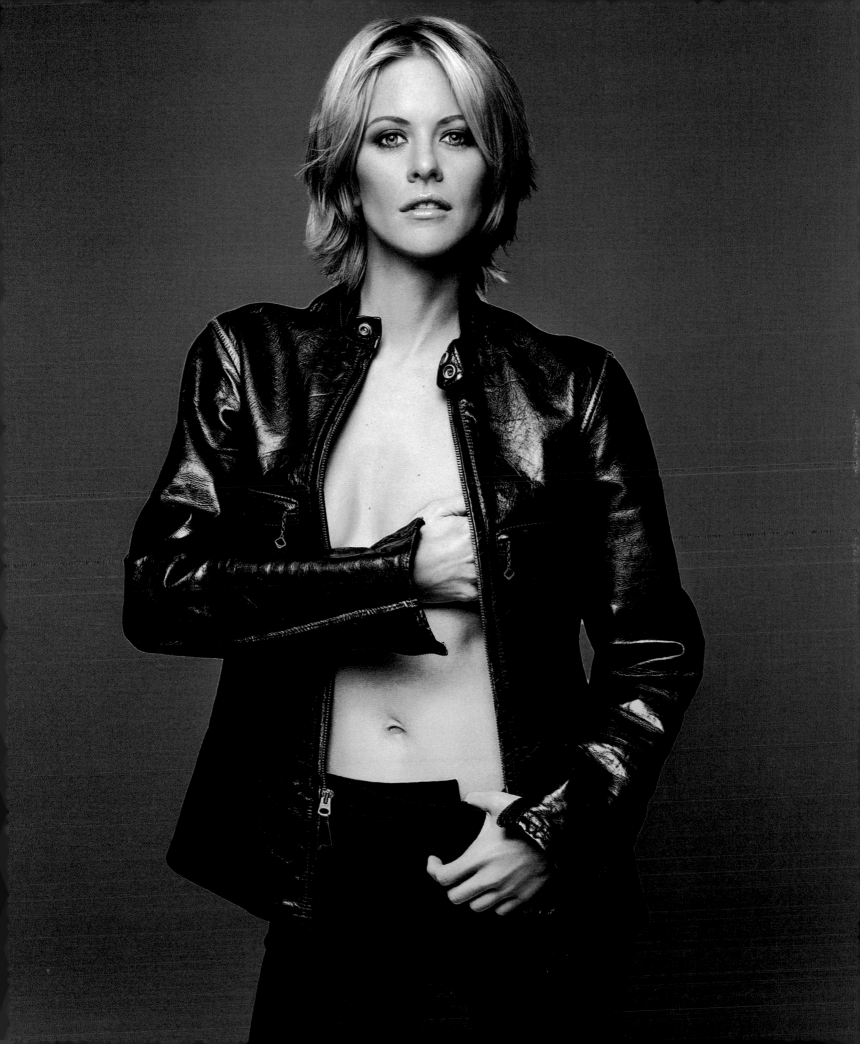

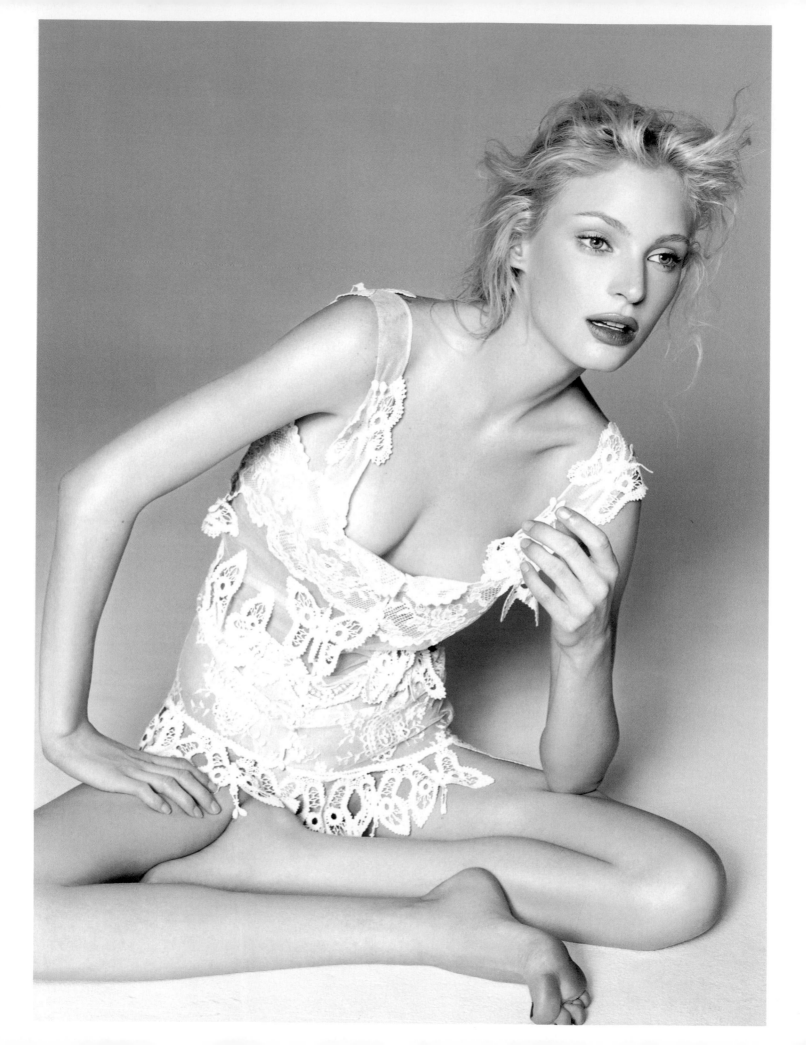

When layering products with SPF, remember that you can't accumulate sunscreen protection. If you're wearing a moisturizer with SPF 15 and foundation with SPF 8*, that's terrific, but together they don't equal SPF 22. If you want a higher SPF, you'll have to wear something with a higher SPF. Also, SPF is an indicator of how long you can stay in the sun, not the strength of the protection.

*Almost all foundations have a minimum of SPF 8 because of the pigments.

beauty secret > Treat your hands the same way you treat your face. They are a tell-tale sign of a woman's age, and if neglected, can make you seem older than you are. Exfoliate and moisturize them regularly. I always forget to wear gloves when I'm working around my house or my garden, but they're an excellent way to protect your hands from cleaning products and water. I'm going to try to make this a habit!

Fake Your Suntan

Self-tanners are so advanced these days, you don't need the sun to look as if you spent a week on the French Riviera. Now you can be tan and have younger-looking skin at the same time. Although the orangey formulas of my youth are long

See how beautiful pale skin can be. Amy Wesson by Michael Thompson.

gone, some women can wind up a little too yellow or orange if they don't apply their self-tanner correctly. First, make sure the formula is right for your skin tone. If you're pale, start with a formula for light skin, no matter how deep and dark you want your tan to be. Before application, make sure you scrub with an exfoliant from head to toe, especially on those areas where the product tends to collect: your knuckles, knees, elbows, ankles, and feet.

The newest products on the market combine moisturizer and self-tanner for easy application. (The labels say things like "gradual glow" or "build your tan.") If you're a self-tan novice, try these first because mistakes are practically invisible. Once you get the hang of it, move on to the stronger stuff.

Exfoliate Your Skin

Whether you're self-tanning or not, scrubs are great for certain skin types. They're a terrific way to exfoliate your skin and boost circulation. How frequently you scrub depends on your skin. My skin is a light olive tone and very normal, so I can exfoliate every morning, which I do in the shower when my pores are open. If your skin is delicate, sensitive, or prone to breakouts, you shouldn't scrub too often. Do it gently and only in key areas that need exfoliation.

A scrub should never hurt or feel abrasive. It should feel invigorating. If you're exfoliating your face, make sure you're using a scrub specially formulated for your complexion.

Facial Facts

I'll talk more about masks in Chapter 9, Groomed and Gorgeous, but it's worth mentioning that they're a great way to pamper and treat your skin, whether you give yourself a quick mask or get a professional facial. I barely have time for facials, but I try to do a mask once a week. The secret is not making a big production of it. Sometimes I leave it on for five minutes or fifteen minutes; other times I wear one in the shower or in the bath. The mask I choose depends on the climate, the time of year, and how my skin is feeling. It's important to listen to your skin. I simply love clay masks in the summer and hydrating masks in the winter.

Professional facials are wonderful if you have the time and the money. Just make sure you're clear on what you want and what you are getting. Some facials include microdermabrasion, which is fine a few times a year and as long as you don't have sensitive skin. Your aesthetician might do extractions, which involve removing black heads from your skin and can be slightly painful. You shouldn't have any red marks when you leave, but sometimes you do. These red marks can take several days to heal, so keep that in mind and try not to schedule a facial before an important event.

Actually, don't try anything new regarding your face right before a big event, like a wedding, reunion, prom, or business presentation. This is a good rule to follow. If you've got one of these events coming up, and you've never had a glycolic peel or microdermabrasion or used a certain antiaging product, then postpone it for after the event. Also, make sure your aesthetician comes highly recommended. Skills vary from facialist to facialist, so investigate before you trust someone with your face.

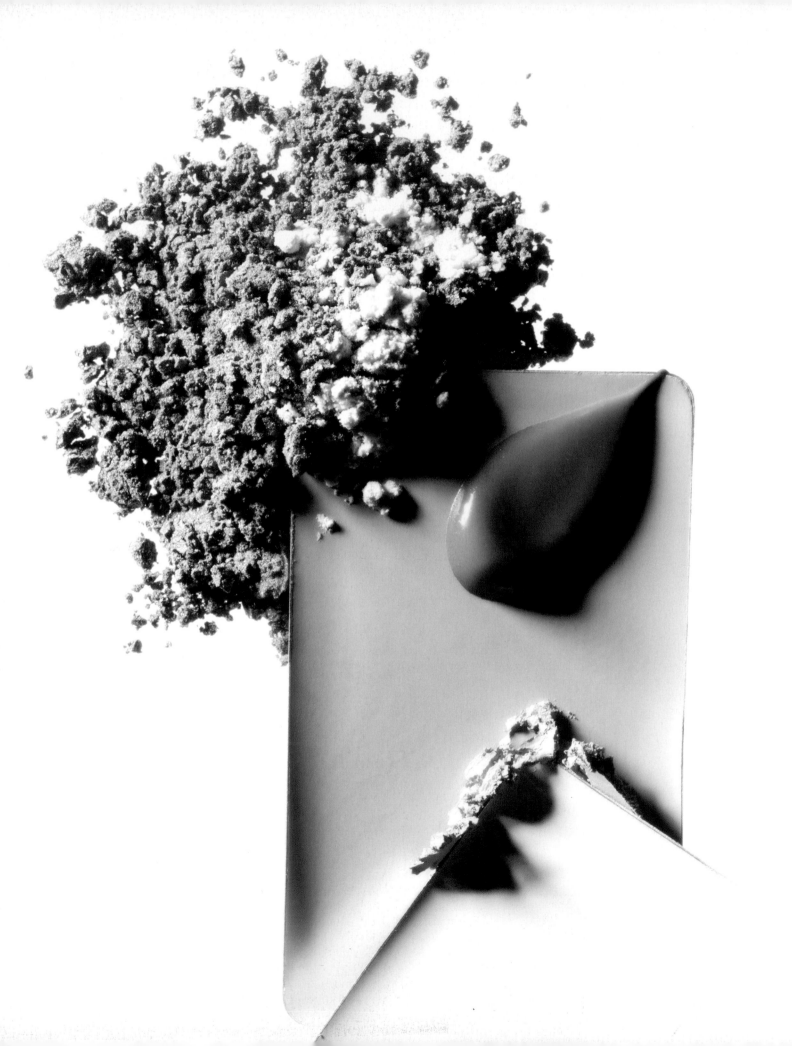

chapter five the flawless face

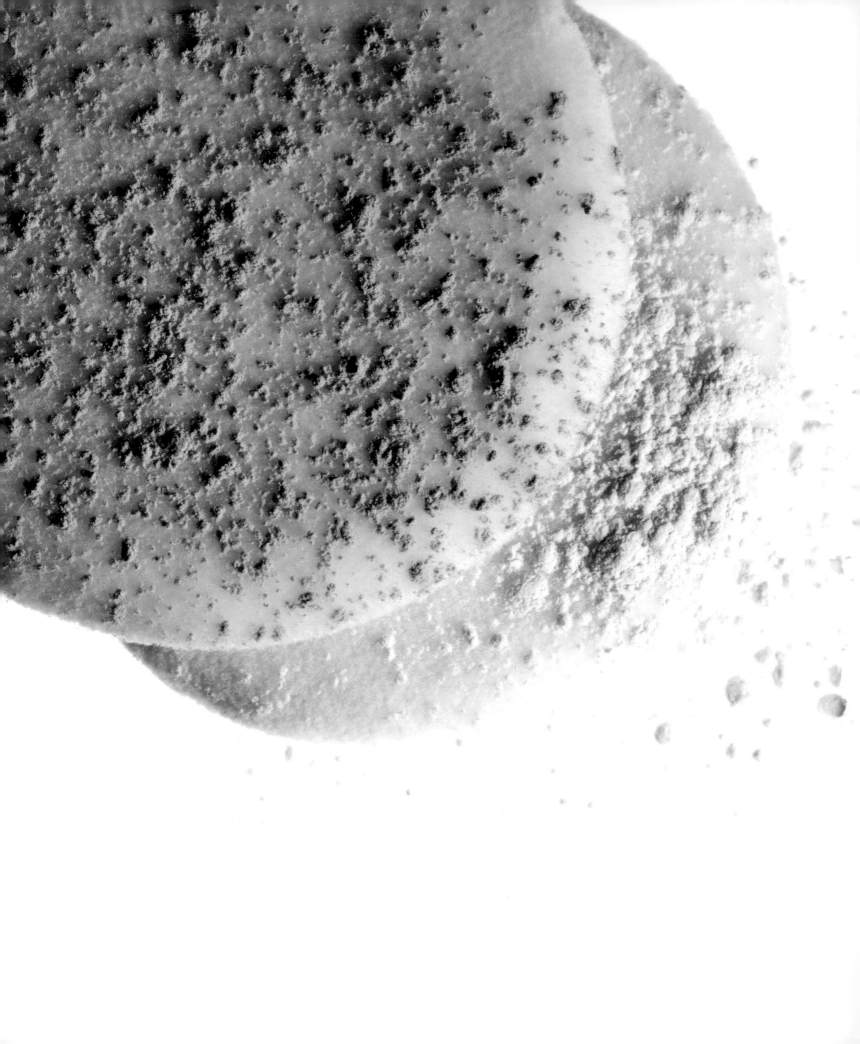

Don't be scared by the word *flawless*. In this case, it's not synonymous with naturally perfect, blemish-free skin, nor with heavy makeup and an hour of application time. *The Flawless Face* is a technique I developed early in my career for making skin look as radiant and perfect as it can be—using as little makeup as possible.

The Flawless Face process can involve any or all of the following basic products:

1   Primer

2   Foundation

3   Concealer

4   Camouflage

5   Loose translucent powder

It's not necessary to use all of these. If you're blessed with good skin, for example, some concealer and powder may suffice. If you need your makeup to last all day at work or you have skin issues to cover up, you'll need more makeup. Basically, you should wear the amount with which you're comfortable. If that means no makeup, so be it. If that means a face full of products, that's fine too. I'll teach you how to do it so that people see you, not the makeup.

I've refined *The Flawless Face* system throughout the years by working on thousands of different women. I've watched how makeup lasts on a model's face at a studio or outdoors during an all-day fashion shoot. I've seen how *The Flawless Face* photographs on an actress walking the red carpet of an awards ceremony. And I've seen how it works under the fluorescent lights of a department store counter as I've taught women how to do makeup that is beautiful and long-lasting. In this chapter, I'm going to teach you how to do *The Flawless Face* on your own with minimum fuss and maximum results.

Skincare Counts

As we discussed in the previous chapter, good skincare and great looking makeup go hand in hand. However, if you have skin problems, don't despair. A solid skincare regimen and a good diet should result in some improvement; if they don't or it's not happening quickly enough, I've got plenty of tips for hiding the things you'd like to cover.

Concealer Versus Camouflage

What's the difference between these two products? Concealer is something creamy and emollient that you use under your eyes to conceal discoloration and dark circles. It's designed to work with the very delicate skin in that area. Camouflage has a much drier consistency and is designed to hide pimples, redness, veins, broken capillaries, sunspots, and other such issues on your face. Although everyone thinks concealer can be used for anything, that's not true. If you use concealer and camouflage the way I suggest, you'll get better results.

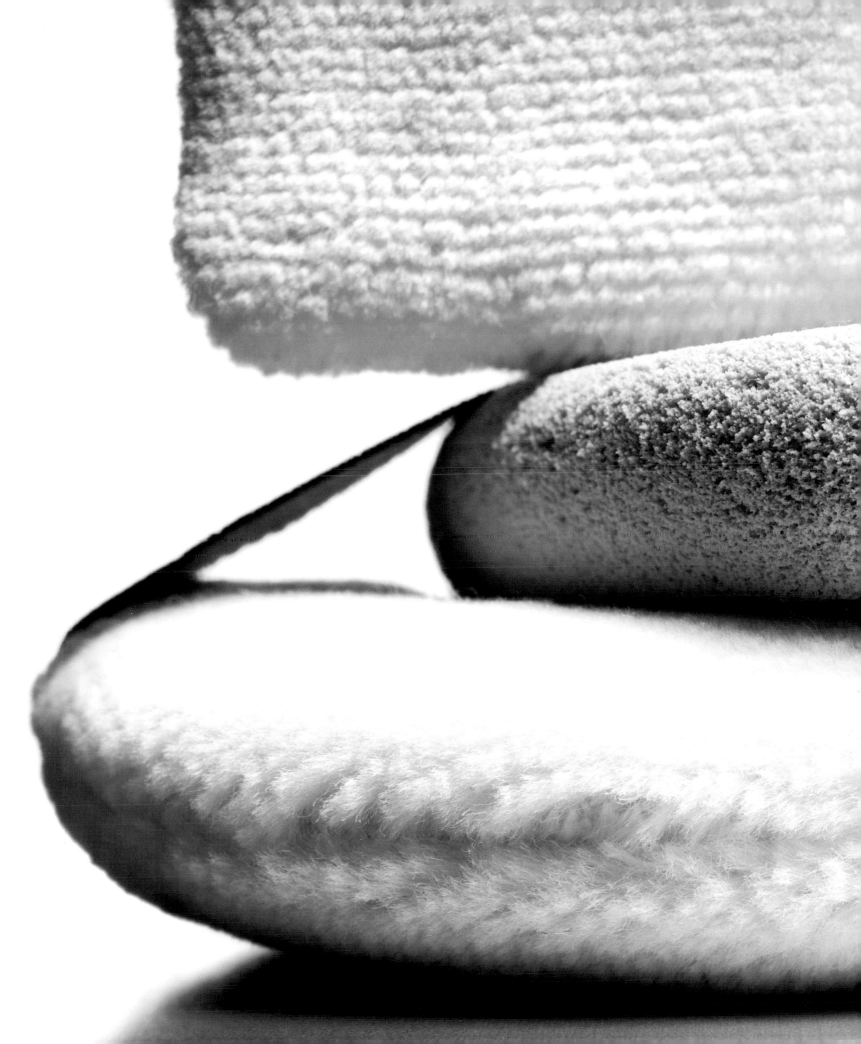

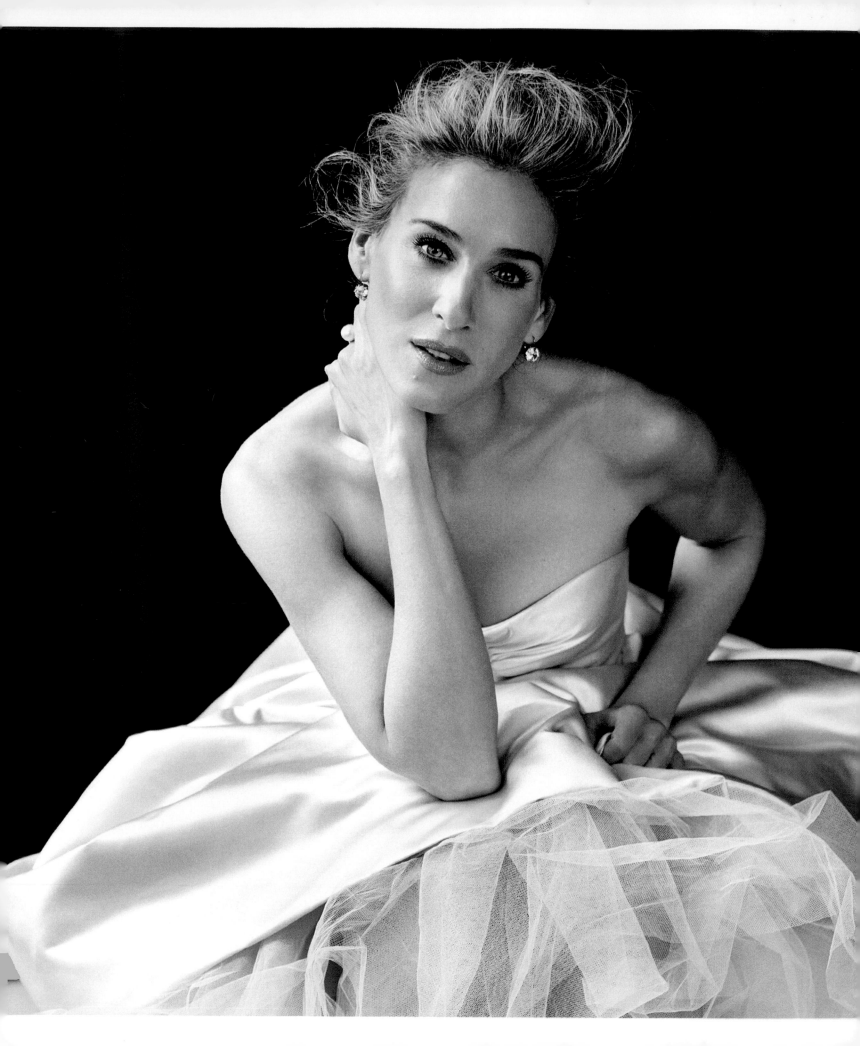

Getting Started

The Recommended Tools

Egg-shaped makeup sponges

Concealer/camouflage brush

Small powder brush

Powder puff

And, of course, *clean hands!* Don't even think about touching

your face with dirty hands.

Primed and Ready

Primer is a fairly misunderstood product. Most women skip using it because they don't know what it is or what it does. A serum-like gel, primer seals in your moisturizer and provides a smooth surface for foundation. It's similar to the primer used to fill imperfections on a wall before a coat of paint is applied.

Primer also keeps your cosmetics from being absorbed into the skin, giving your makeup greater staying power throughout the day.

Sarah Jessica Parker by Michael Thompson in the ad for her fragrance Lovely

How to Apply

If you're going to wear foundation or powder, primer is a must. Put a quarter-size amount in your palm, spread it over your fingers and gently massage the product over your entire face, just as you would moisturizer. Avoid your eyelids if the skin there tends to be sensitive. If you can tolerate primer, it's great for your eye makeup.

Cover Your Bases

Foundation is next. Many women think foundation is meant to cover imperfections, so they tend to use too much, resulting in a cakey or masklike texture. Foundation's only purpose is to

> beauty secret > If you're prone to puffiness or live in a warm climate, keep your makeup primer in your refrigerator to instantly calm and cool your face.

even out your skin tone. Don't use it to erase every pore and hide every freckle.

If you need foundation, it's worth taking the time to find the right one. There are so many different formulas available today that it's mind-boggling. Do you want oil-free, moisturizing, or long-lasting? Think about your skin's needs and select the formula that makes sense. Then determine the amount of coverage you want—sheer, medium, or heavy. If your skin is fairly even, go for the lighter option; if your complexion is not very even, you'll want more coverage. The amount of coverage depends on the amount of pigment; the more pigment a foundation contains, the heavier it's going to feel. (If you buy a foundation that's too pigmented or heavy, you can make it sheer by applying it with a damp sponge.)

Elizabeth Hurley, the great Estée Lauder spokesmodel and British beauty. Photo by Michael Thompson.

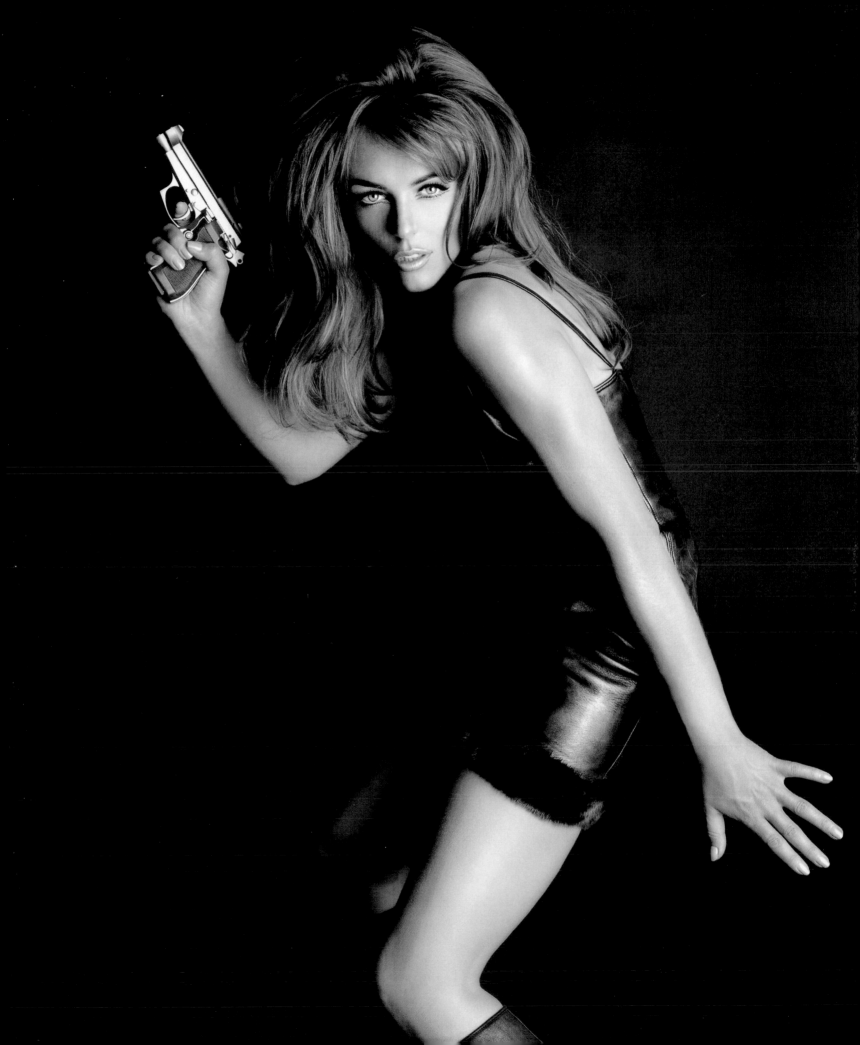

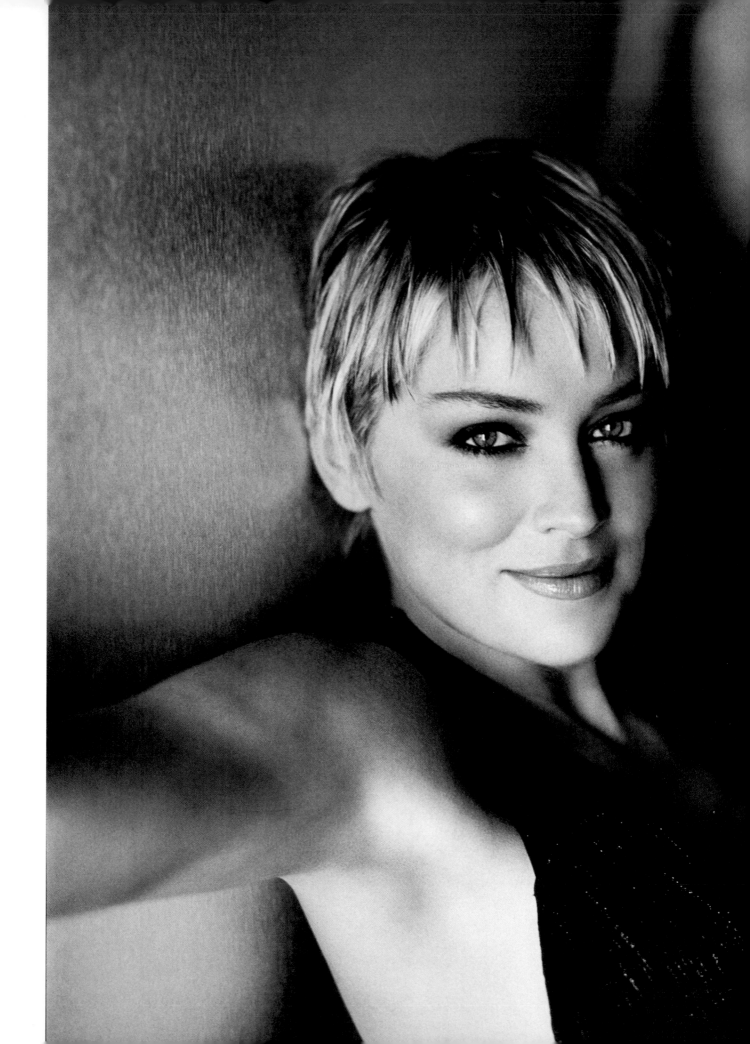

Nobody can do base makeup like Laura does.

I'm great at putting my makeup on—but you need

a real makeup artist to do your base.

—Sharon Stone

As for the delivery system, you have liquid, cream, or stick formulations. The tips I discuss below refer to liquid foundation, but you can adapt the information for stick or cream.

Color Selection

To be sure you've got the perfect shade for you, pick three colors from the same range that are closest to your complexion tone. Put a small stripe of each on the skin right above your jaw line. The one that seems to disappear is the best foundation for you.

beauty secret > Don't test foundation on the back of your hand. It's a simple way to see what a color looks like, but the skin there is very different from the skin on your face. Apply it right on your cheek. Remember, the perfect color should practically disappear.

If the skin tone on your face, neck, and chest don't match, you may have to adjust your foundation for that. Probably 85 percent of the Laura Mercier users I have met have face, neck, and chest skin colors that don't match. You can bring all the tones in line by blending a darker tinted moisturizer into your foundation so your face can match a darker décolletage, for example. You can do this trick in the summer if you get a little sun and your foundation is too light or if you protect your face but get some color on your chest.

Make sure your foundation isn't too pink or too yellow. Sometimes, in an attempt to look natural, women with pink or red skin tones will gravitate toward pink formulas and women with yellow, olive, or sallow skin will gravitate toward yellow. Look for a color that is more balanced; otherwise, you'll just overemphasize the undertone.

How to Apply

I love using a cosmetics sponge for an even application of product. You can use a dry sponge or a slightly damp one for sheer application. Just moisten the sponge, and squeeze out any excess water. Either way, place a small amount of foundation in the palm of your clean hand, work the product into the narrow end of the sponge and smooth lightly and evenly over your face. Most of the time, I recommend avoiding the eye area. You don't want to bring a lot of texture underneath the eyes, especially if you have darkness or wrinkles, and you're going to use a concealer there next. The more texture from makeup you put there, the more you emphasize any lines.

I always apply foundation from the outer portion of the face in toward the nose. If you start in the center of your face, you usually put too much texture around the mouth and nose. Your foundation should never stop at your jaw line, so work it below your jaw with the sponge and blend well.

A Hint of Tint

If you're not a fan of foundation, but need to even your skin tone a little, try a tinted moisturizer. This product tends to be very natural looking and slightly dewy. You can use it alone (apply in the same manner as you apply moisturizer) or in conjunction with concealer, camouflage, and powder.

Concealer Basics

As we discussed earlier, concealer is used exclusively under your eyes to cover dark circles and brighten shadows. The formula you choose needs to provide coverage, so skip the sheer, liquidy concealers that don't do much of anything. Your concealer also needs to be supple and hydrating, since the skin under your eyes tends to be drier and thinner than elsewhere on your face.

Some people can get away with no foundation, but I find most of them benefit from concealer.

The Right Color

You want your concealer to be light enough to brighten the eye area and conceal your undereye circles, yet not so light that it doesn't blend nicely with your skin tone. Make sure to avoid raccoon eyes, where the undereye area is noticeably lighter than the rest of your face.

Use the color and tone of your undereye area as a guide to finding the best concealer color. If your undereye area is blue or purple, then try warm beige-tone concealer. If your undereye area is yellow, green, or brown, then try pinkish beige-tone concealer.

In some cases, there is puffiness under the eye that is white. In that case, you'd want a darker-tone concealer to recede the puffiness.

Sarah Jessica Parker as Sarah Bernhardt by Laspata DeCaro

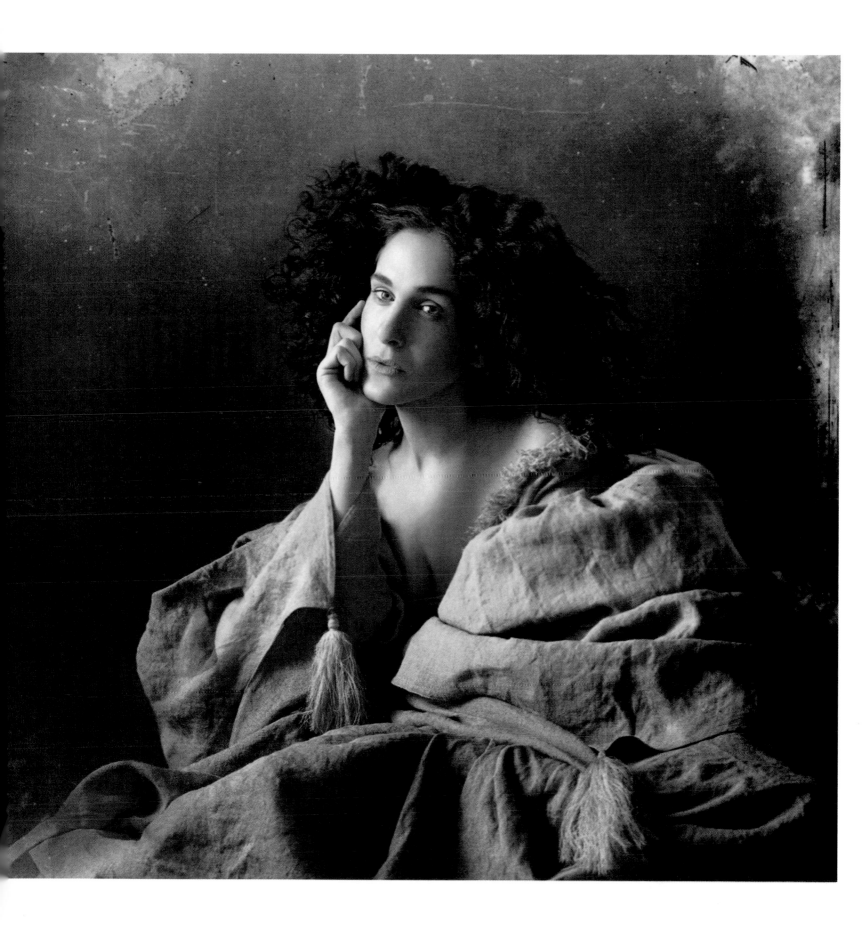

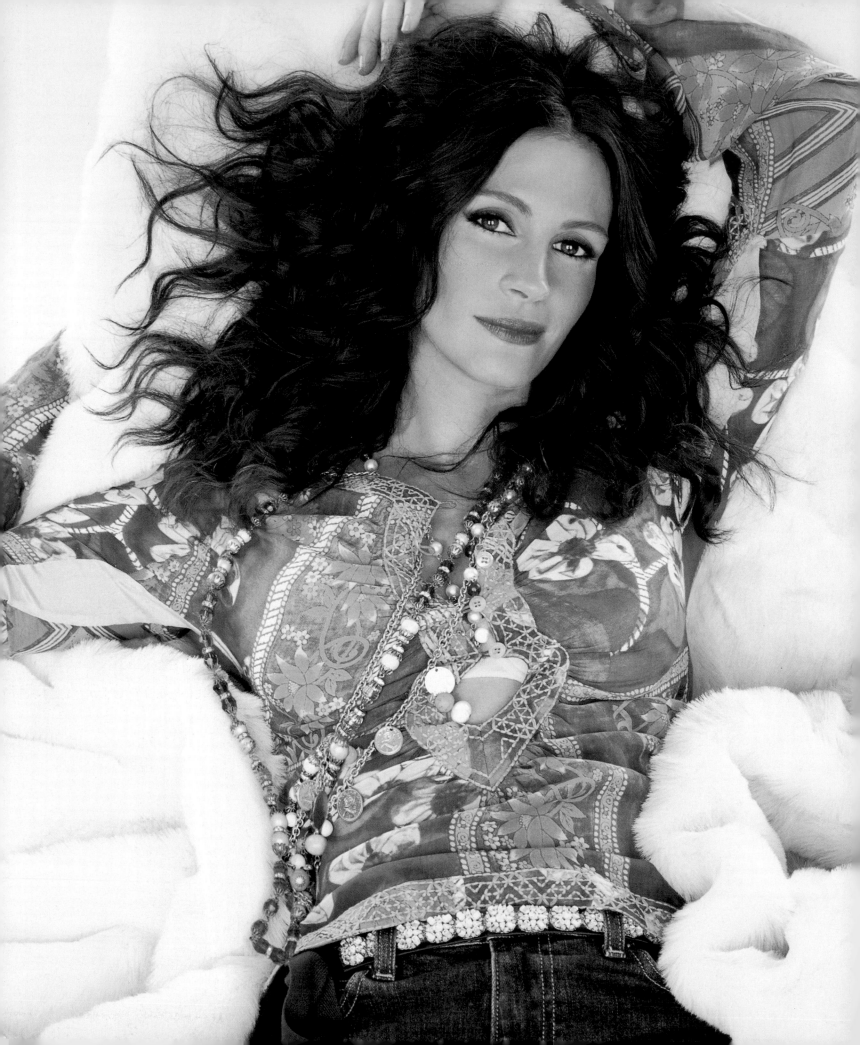

How to Apply

Put some concealer on the back of your hand, using your hand like a painter's palette, to control the amount on your brush. (If you're mixing two shades, then do so now. Once the concealer is mixed, wipe the brush on the back of your hand to remove excess product.) You don't want too much product on the brush. Multiple applications of light coats result in better, more natural-looking coverage. Applying too much at once results in obvious texture. Apply to the dark undereye areas, including the inner and outer corners of your eyes. If the skin under your lashline is dark or reddish, you can apply concealer there as well, but avoid this step if you don't need it. You'll just build too much unnecessary texture.

Covering Large Circles

If you have a large, dark, and flat area to cover with concealer, you can use your finger. Apply by gently blending the product over the area, so the darkness is cancelled out but brightened.

Setting Your Concealer

You need to set your concealer right after you've applied it and *before* you apply camouflage and powder to the rest of your face. Don't set the rest of the face before setting your concealer.

Julia Roberts, radiant and serene. Photo by Michael Thompson.

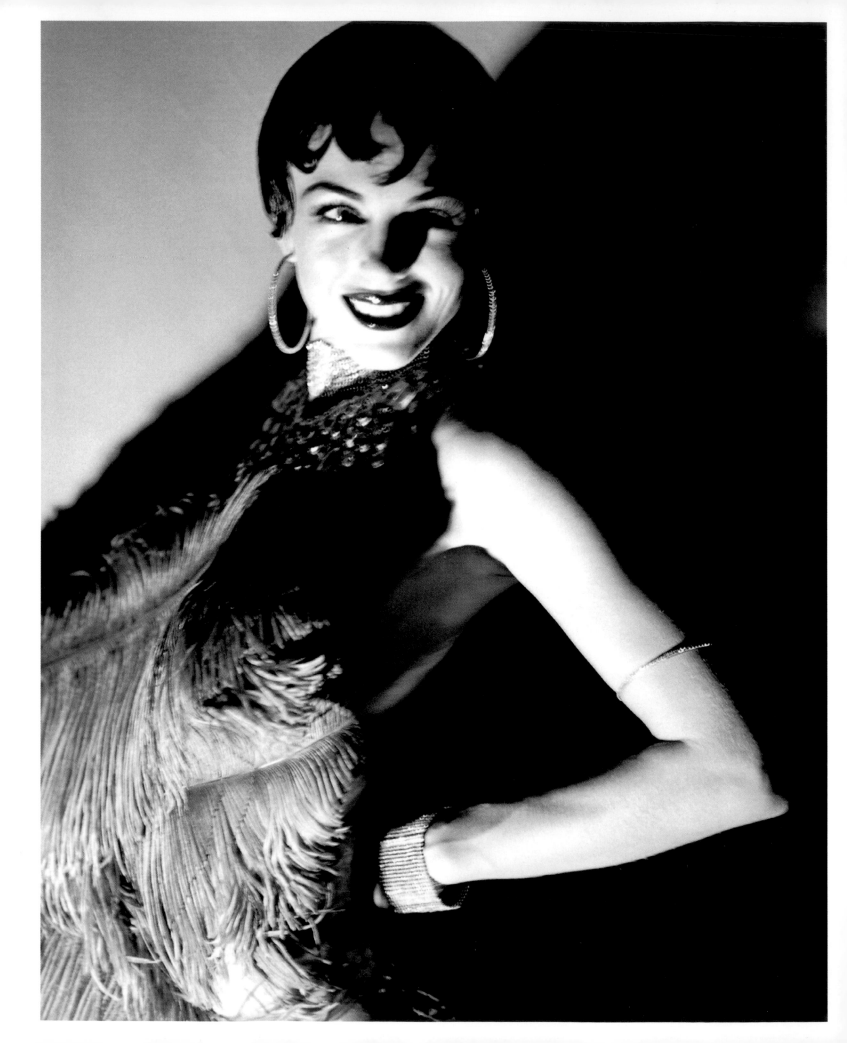

I prefer to use a special brightening powder and apply it under the eyes with a small powder setting brush. Put a tiny bit of powder on the side of the brush, and press gently over the concealer. Don't drag the brush. Keep pressing it against your skin gently until you've covered the area and the skin feels soft and silky to the touch. You can use a puff and basic translucent powder if you don't want to add more products and tools to your routine, but you will have less control over the amount of powder you apply.

Extra Help

If your undereye area needs more of a boost than concealer can provide, then try a highlighting cream underneath. This gel-like formula comes in an applicator pen with a built-in brush, and it reinforces the light-reflecting quality of your concealer. Just pump the pen to dispense the liquid and apply after your eye cream. You can layer your concealer right on top of the highlighting cream then set with the translucent or brightening powder.

The Cover-up

If you have any pimples, age spots, shadows, scars, or redness to cover, this is where your camouflage product comes in. Camouflage is more pigmented than concealer, and it's less emollient so it won't slide around. Look for camouflage that's formulated for troubled skin so it's ok to put on top of pimples.

How to Apply

The application process for camouflage depends on the size of the area you are covering. For small areas and spots, use a special concealer/camouflage brush. (Make sure to wipe off the brush first after using it for concealer.) As with concealer, put some camouflage on the back of your hand and move it around with the brush to warm the product for easy application. (If you're mixing two colors, then do so now.) Once the camouflage is warmed and mixed, wipe the bristles on the back of your hand to remove excess product. You want only a little product on the brush. Applying too much at once results in too much texture that is difficult to remove. Several light applications are better than too much product at once. Remember, it's a building process. If you're going to cover a pimple, spot, or vein, use the tip of the brush. Dot or draw on it as delicately and precisely as possible. Repeat as necessary. For medium-size areas, you can use the side of the brush.

beauty secret > Can't find the right camouflage or concealer shade for your complexion? You may need to mix two shades together. Some products come with two or three colors in one compact so you can customize; in other cases, you may need to buy two shades.

Don't get discouraged. The more you practice, the better you'll become at this technique. Everyone tends to be too heavy handed the first few times.

For large areas, use your finger. This works if you need to cover any rosacea, red patches, or dark pigmentation. Warm the product on the back of your hand, then

Shalom Harlow by Miles Aldridge

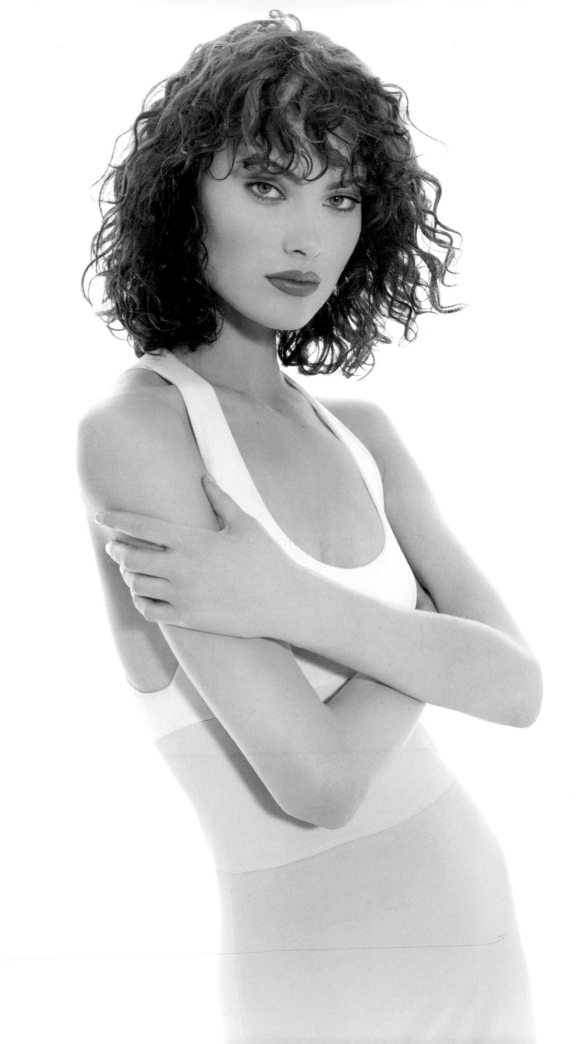

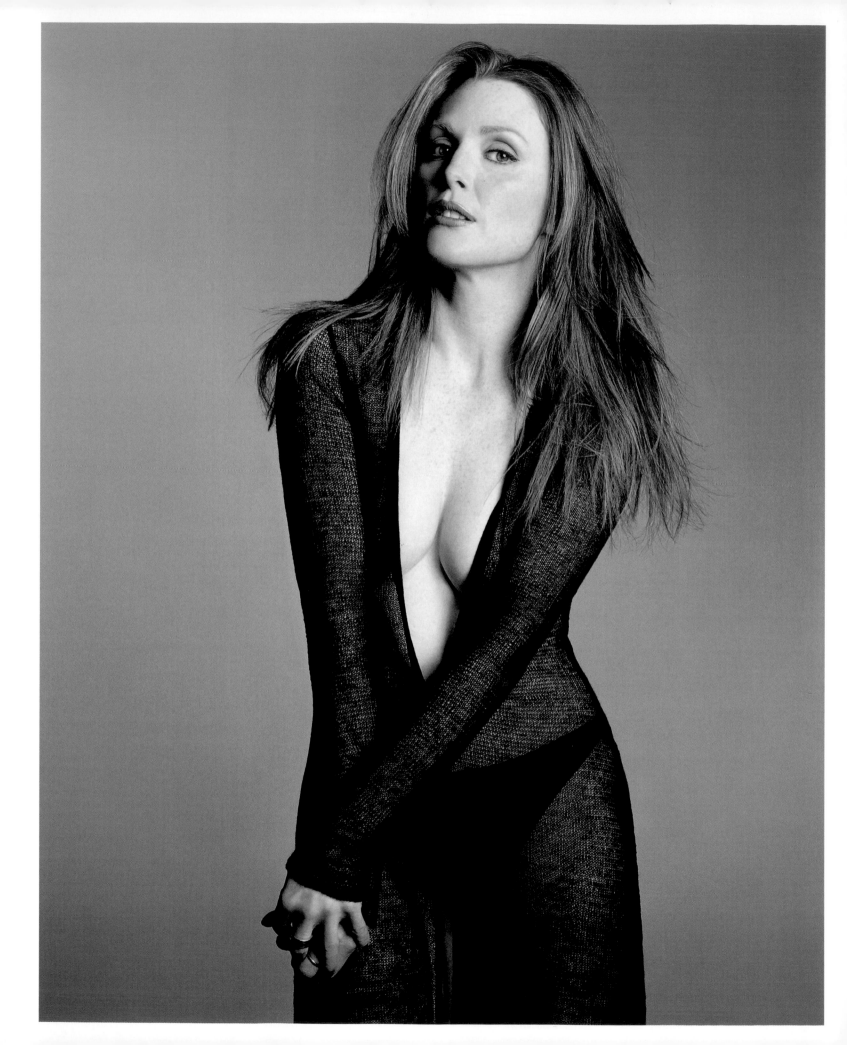

apply by gently pushing the product into your pores with your finger. (Never spread your camouflage with your finger. You'll apply too much. Pushing leaves a lighter coat by making the product melt invisibly into the skin.) Again, multiple light coats as a building technique are preferable to a heavy application all at once.

Powder Makes Perfect

Loose translucent powder is the finishing touch for *The Flawless Face*. Powder? *Oui!* If you're not a fan, I know what you're thinking. It's old fashioned, it's leftover from the eighties when faces were totally matte, or it's not the look you want.

Translucent powder isn't meant to erase every bit of glow from your face. When applied properly, it's a product that sets the makeup underneath and helps your foundation, concealer, and camouflage stay in place. It also preps the face for any colored powder cosmetics that will follow, such as powder blush or bronzer. Without that fine layer of translucent powder, the colored pigments will grab onto moisture or dry patches and look blotchy.

Julianne Moore by Michael Thompson

What Is Translucent Powder?

It's a pigment-free powder that can be used on any skin tone because it literally disappears once applied. True translucent powder should not turn ashy on darker skin tones. I use loose translucent powder for the initial *Flawless Face* steps, as opposed to pressed translucent powder, which is the kind you find in a compact. Pressed powder is fine for touchups through the day, but it tends to go on slightly heavier than loose powder.

Women with darker skin tones need a completely translucent powder that happens to be white. That means absolutely no pigment has been used to color the powder, and you won't get that ashiness that results from light pigments. If you have dark skin and feel more comfortable using a dark powder that matches your skin tone, apply a fine layer of translucent powder first and the darker powder on top. This way, the colored pigments will go on evenly.

Light as Air

When buying powder, touch it first and make sure it feels smooth and silky. Put some on the back of your hand to see if it looks sheer and natural on your skin. Otherwise, you may end up with something that looks too chalky.

Forget about dipping a large fluffy brush into your powder and sweeping it all over your face. It may be the way you've always seen it applied, but I personally don't like that technique for applying translucent powder. It doesn't result in a fine, even application, and it can disrupt the product underneath. (Use a large powder brush to build coverage with a colored powder after the setting process.)

Here's how to do the setting process. Spill a bit of loose translucent powder into the lid of the jar. Take a velour powder puff, and fold it in half so that your finger is in the middle. Dip it into the powder, and tap the powdered side of the puff against the back of your hand to work the powder into the puff, and get rid of the excess. You will leave a powdery residue each time you press the puff against your hand. Continue to do so until the residue no longer appears. Now the puff is ready for your face.

Gently press the puff, which should still be folded around your finger, against your face, roll, and lift. Continue to press, roll, and lift the puff on your entire face. You don't want to use too much powder, but don't underdo it either. Use enough powder so that your skin feels silky to the touch. Your face will look slightly matte, but if you've applied the right amount, a slight glow will soon return to your face.

Powder your cheeks if you plan to apply powder blush. If you've applied cream blush and want to keep the glow, leave unpowdered. As for your undereye area, you should have already set your concealer, so don't powder this area again.

Powder Foundation

If you have acne, rosacea, or discoloration and want additional coverage, powder foundation can help. Use a large powder brush to apply. Tap off any excess, and apply right on top of your translucent powder. The powder foundation fills in depressions and adds a velvety covering where you need it.

Bronze Goddess

Everybody needs to feel a little St. Tropez fabulous from time to time, and nothing does the trick like bronzer. It's so easy to use, but it's an intimidating product because it

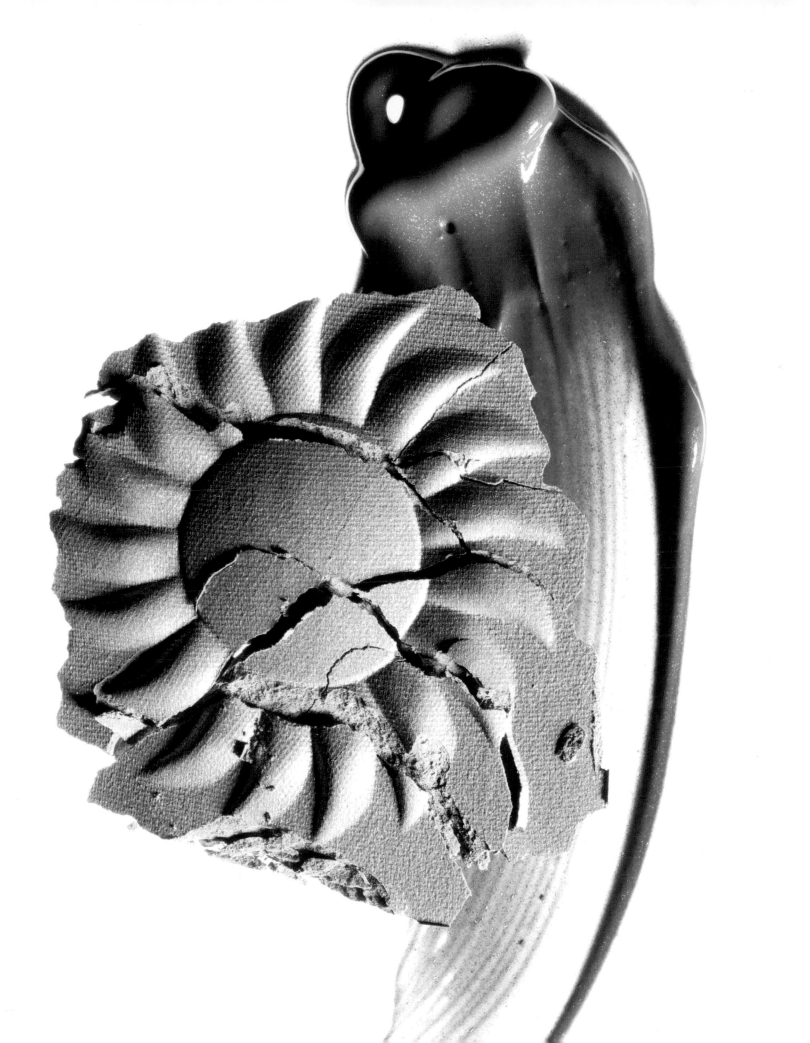

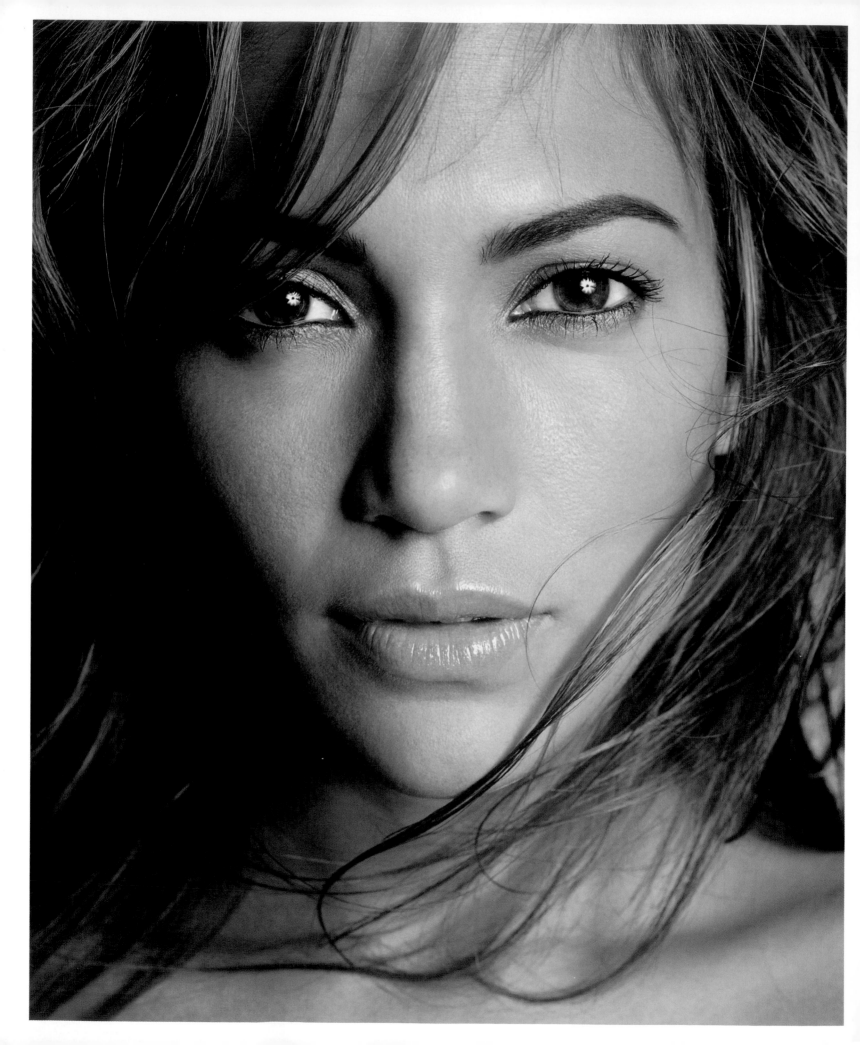

can look fake when applied incorrectly or with a heavy hand. As with foundation, there are several types of bronzers: powder, gel, stick, cream, and liquid.

If you use a powder bronzer, take a large fluffy powder brush and swirl it around the product. Tap off the excess and lightly brush where the sun naturally hits your face: the tops of your cheekbones, tip of your chin, bridge of your nose, and on your forehead at the temples and the hairline. Apply your bronzer before you apply your blush.

The simplest way to go bronze? Add a few drops of liquid bronzer to your foundation and apply.

How to Contour Your Face

You don't need a graduate degree in makeup to contour your face. All you need is a medium-size powder brush and matte bronzer (light for fair skin and dark for darker skin tones). There are special contouring powders and creams on the market, but matte bronzer works just fine because it doesn't contain any light-reflecting ingredients. What you're doing is creating a shadow to distract the eye. Never use blush to contour. It's an old-fashioned way to do it, and it never looks natural.

Jennifer loves a bronzed and beautiful complexion. Photo by Michael Thompson.

Contouring Directions

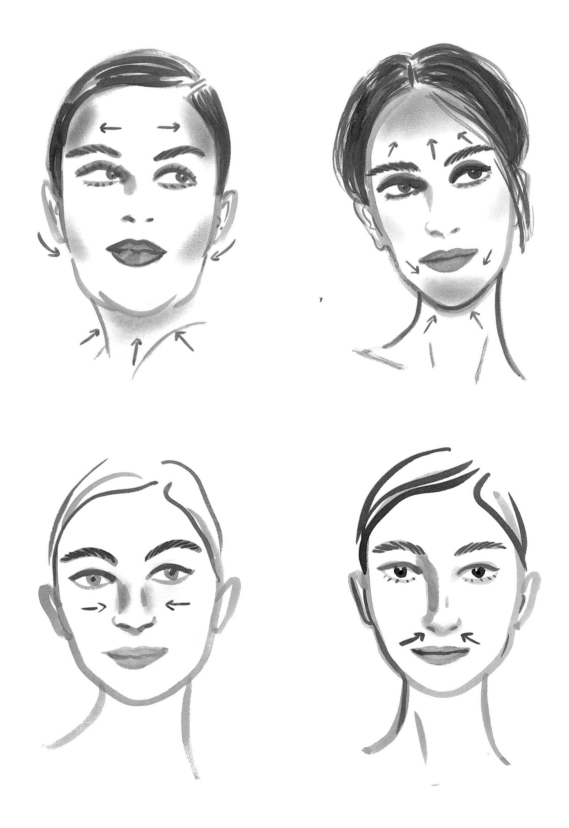

My favorite contouring trick is making a double chin disappear. After you've applied your translucent powder, dip your powder brush into the bronzer, dust off the excess, and apply it right underneath your chin. Be sure to blend well.

Other places to contour are as follows:

Along your jawbone to strengthen its appearance.

On the tip of your nose to shorten it.

Along the sides of your nose to narrow it out.

On the tip of your chin to minimize it.

Under your cheekbones to emphasize them (Don't do this *on* your cheekbones because you'll de-emphasize them).

On the top of your forehead from your hairline down to cut the length of your face.

Au Revoir!

Now that your skin looks better than ever, turn the page and learn how to get a pretty flush worthy of your new complexion.

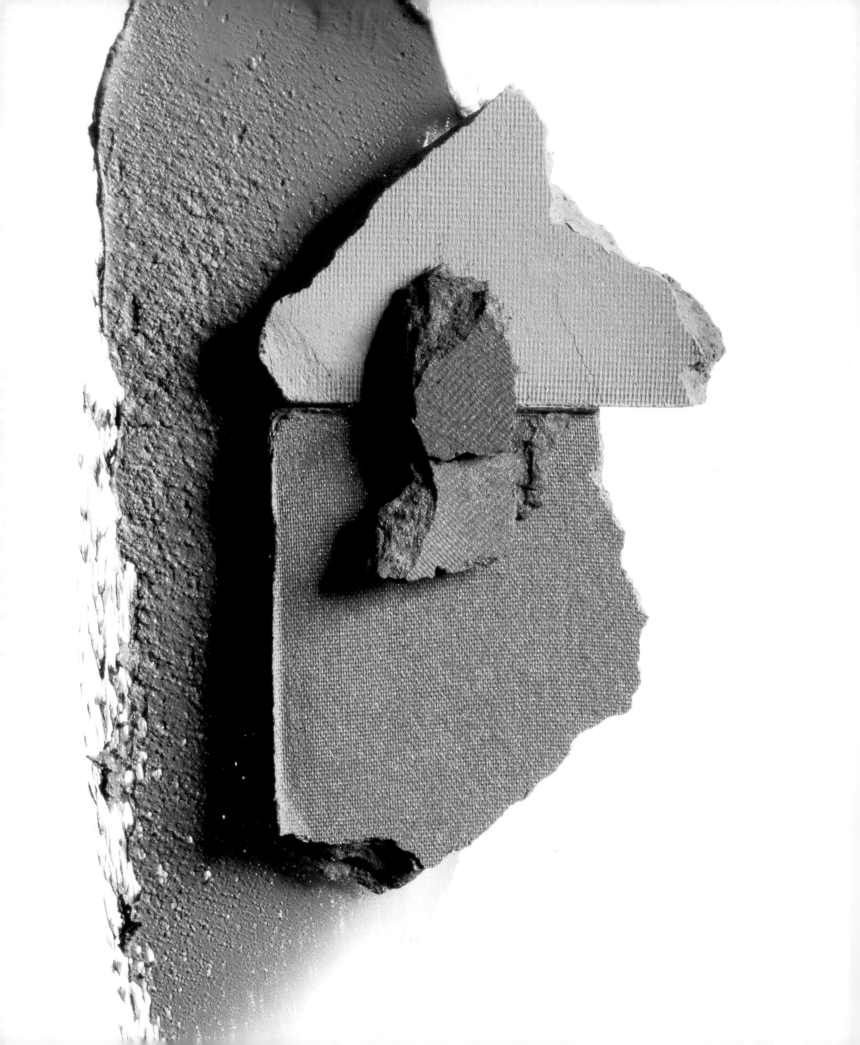

chapter six cheek to cheek

Did you know that Diana Vreeland, the legendary editor in chief of *Vogue* magazine, wore red rouge on her temples, cheeks, and earlobes? She was not bashful about blush, to say the least. Talk about individual! You may not want to steal her look, but you have to admire her spirit. In comparison, my approach to blush is fairly straightforward. Since nothing gives you a sense of youthfulness and the appearance of health the way your cheeks do, I gravitate toward a look that is pretty, natural-looking, and often glowing. After all, the cheeks represent the two largest areas on your face, so they're something people notice.

Beautifully made-up cheeks are an integral component of *The Flawless Face* because they're not an accessory in the way eyes and lips are. Consider them a basic for your face, much in the way a white shirt or a great black jacket complements a brightly colored bag or bold piece of jewelry. Whether I do major eyes and lips or nude eyes and clear gloss, I always apply color to the cheeks, from barely there to fully flushed. If you don't apply any color to your cheeks, then you can look washed out.

The Blush Basics

Cream blush

Cream blush brush (or your fingers!)

Powder blush

Blush brush

Loose powder

Powder puff

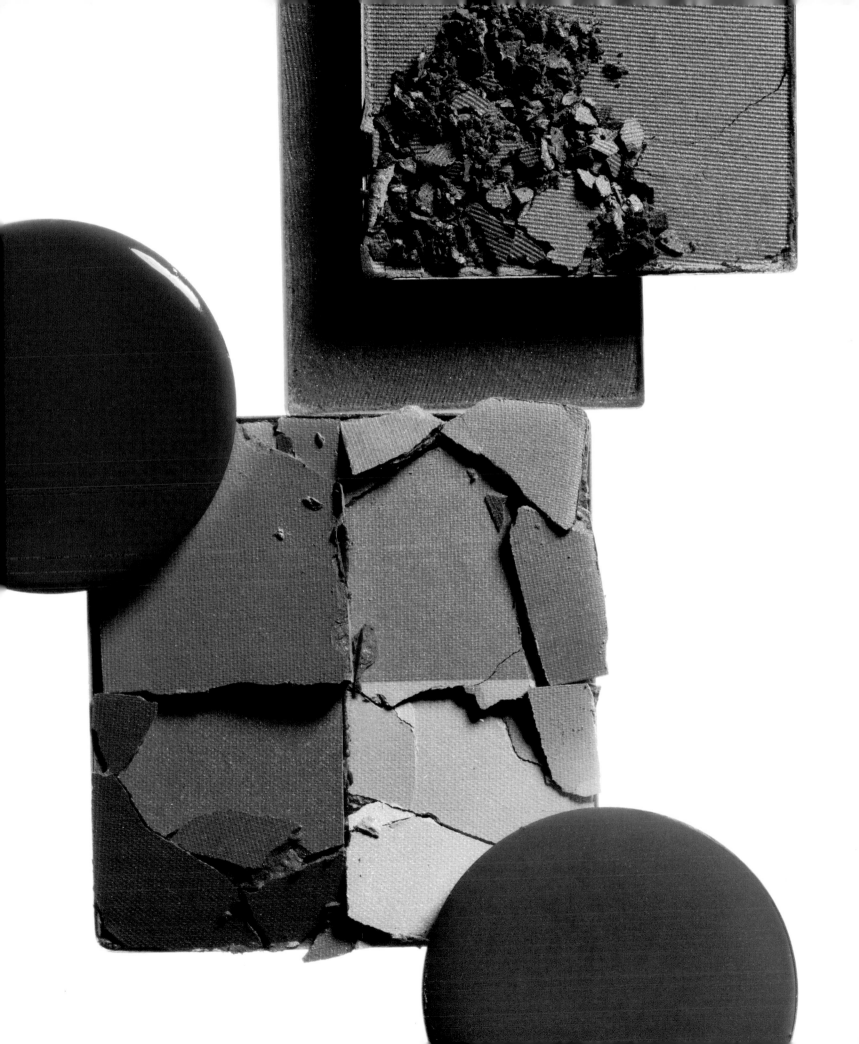

Getting Started

As I mentioned, doing your cheeks is part of *The Flawless Face* process, although we've dedicated a separate chapter to it. I prefer to layer cream blush and powder blush to give the cheeks a bit of dimension and give the color staying power. As you learned in Chapter 5, I apply cream blush after the necessary face products (which include primer, foundation, concealer, and/or camouflage), set everything with a very fine layer of translucent powder, and then apply powder blush. Those are the basic steps, which I'll describe in further detail below. You can adapt this formula to get the look that is right for you.

Choosing the Right Color

Because I favor a natural look with blush, I'm drawn to muted shades such as rose brown, terracotta, apricot, raisin, and crushed berry. Stronger colors look beautiful on darker skin tones.

If you end up with a color that's too bright for you, you can neutralize it with brown or terracotta blush or with bronzer. If the color is too strong, try mixing it with a little translucent powder.

Lara Flynn Boyle with a subtly shaded cheek to complement her other makeup. Photo by Michael Thompson.

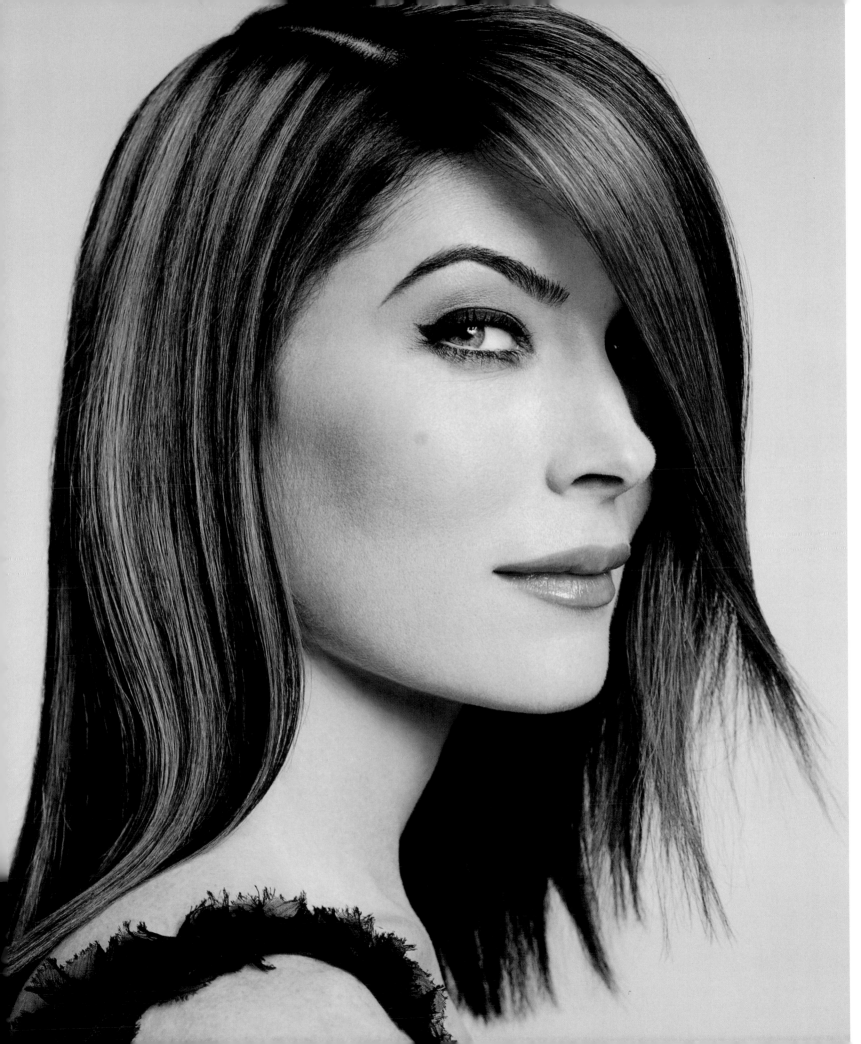

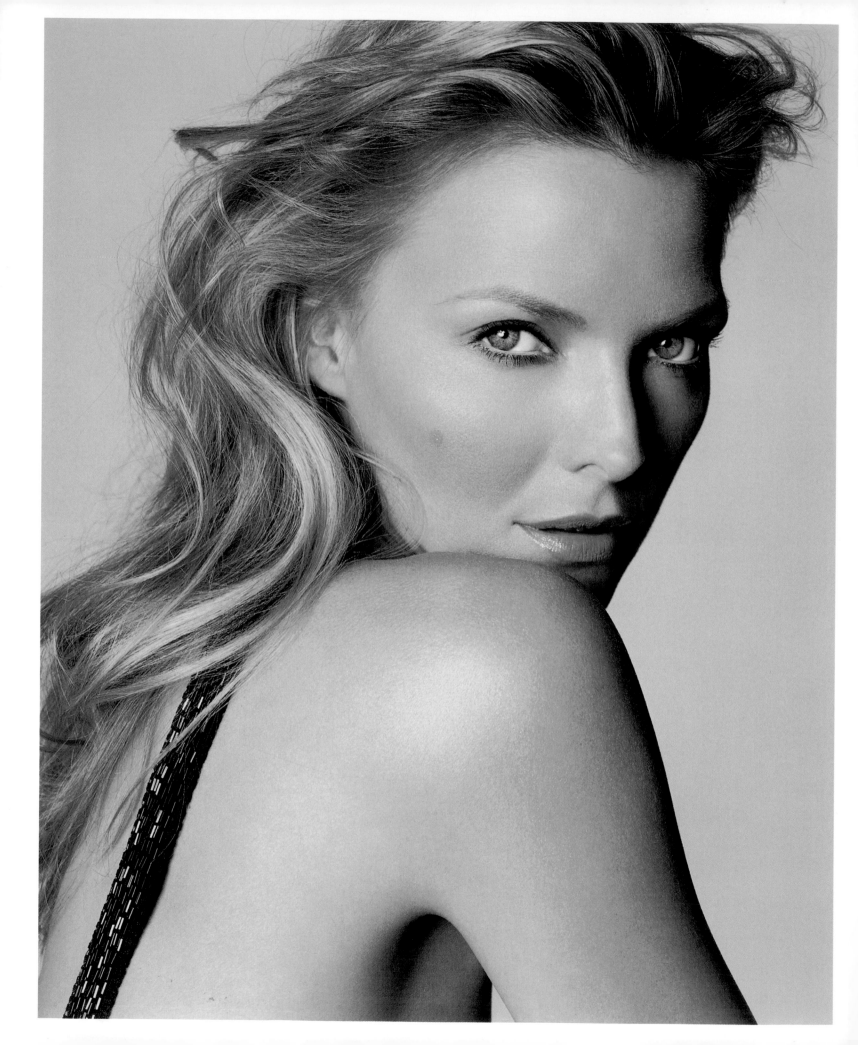

If you're doing a combination of cream and powder blush, the colors don't have to be identical. You can mix and match. Say you really need to brighten your face because you're sallow. Start with a vibrant-colored cream blush because it's easy to blend, and finish with a neutral-tone powder blush. As we've discussed, you never put cream products on top of powder ones. You can leave your cheeks unpowdered for more of a glow, but powdering them will make the color last longer. If you're going to layer your cream and powder blushes, you must apply a layer of translucent powder between them. Whichever step you choose, don't forget to powder the rest of your face to set your foundation, concealer, and/or camouflage.

beauty secret > A cream blush brush is always made of soft, synthetic hair. Remember, natural bristles don't work well with creamy products because they absorb too much of it.

Cream Blush

This is a wonderful product if you want a simple glow because it blends so beautifully—a blessing if you have dry skin, dry patches, or an unevenly textured complexion. It comes in stick form, a pot, or a compact; all three are basically the same in terms of texture. You can apply to naked skin or skin that's been prepared with primer, foundation, or both. Put a few dots of color right on the apples of your cheeks. Blend with your fingers or cream blush brush and *voilà!*

Michelle Pfeiffer in pretty, peachy blush. Photo by Michael Thompson.

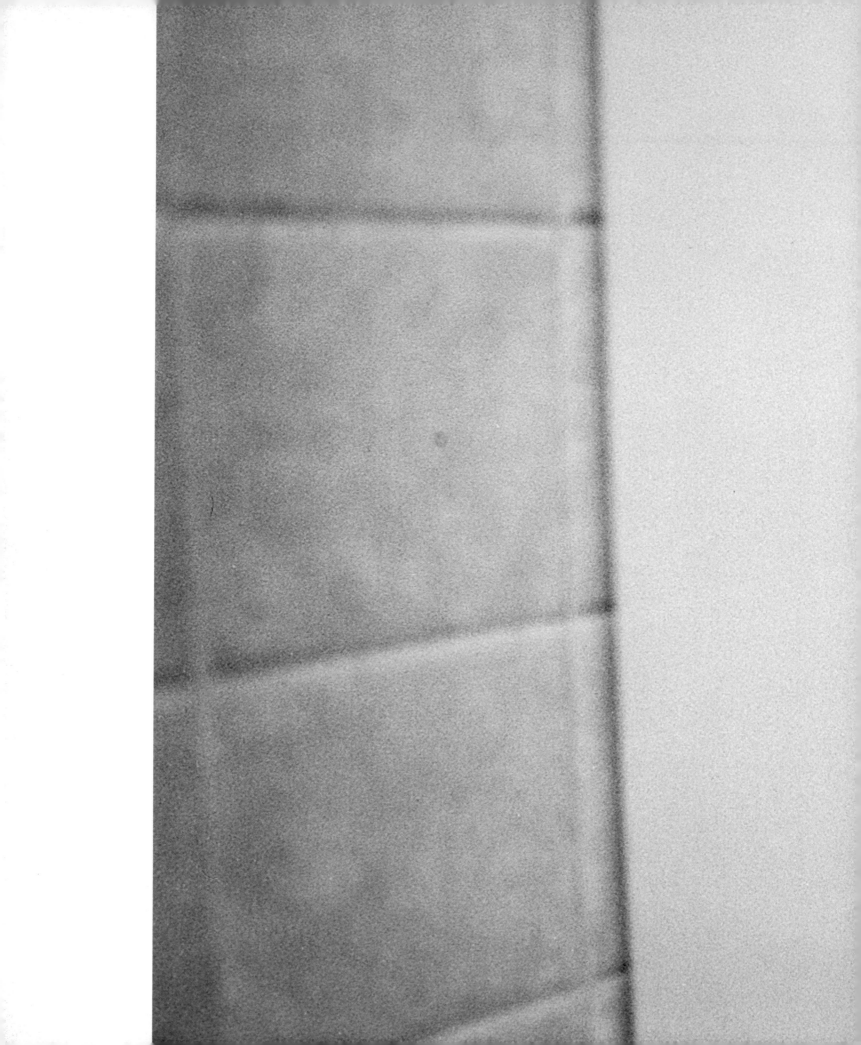

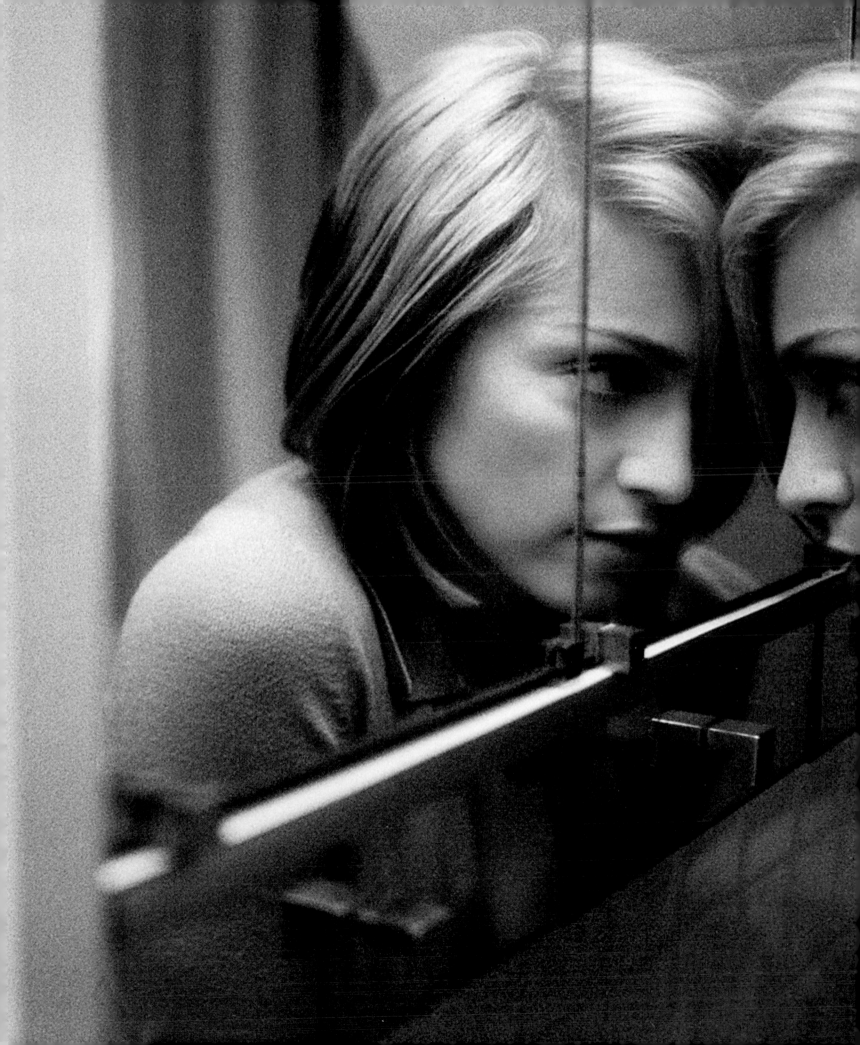

Powder Blush

I have two rules regarding powder blush. You cannot apply it to naked skin because any dry or oily areas are going to grab the pigment of the colored powder, resulting in an uneven application. When the skin has been set with translucent powder, it gives your powder blush a beautiful canvas, so it glides over the surface, depositing color evenly. The second rule is that you cannot apply it directly over creamy products for similar reasons. The dewy areas of your skin will grab the pigment unevenly, resulting in a blotchy look.

beauty secret > Your blush shouldn't be a specific, identifiable shape. Unless you are going for an avant-garde look, you want just a flush of color. No circles, stripes, squares, or checkmarks. Blend well to get a general diffusion of color.

Staying Power (or Staying Powder!)

If your blush tends to fade during the day, try the combination of cream blush, translucent powder, and powder blush. It will last longer and require fewer touch-ups.

Where to Apply

Always start on the apples of your cheeks, whether you're using cream or powder blush. If you're using a brush, then use the sides, not the tops, of the bristles. This gives you more control and lets you build the color gradually, rather than building too much

Previous: Madonna by Glen Luchford
Opposite: Liv Tyler by Michael Thompson

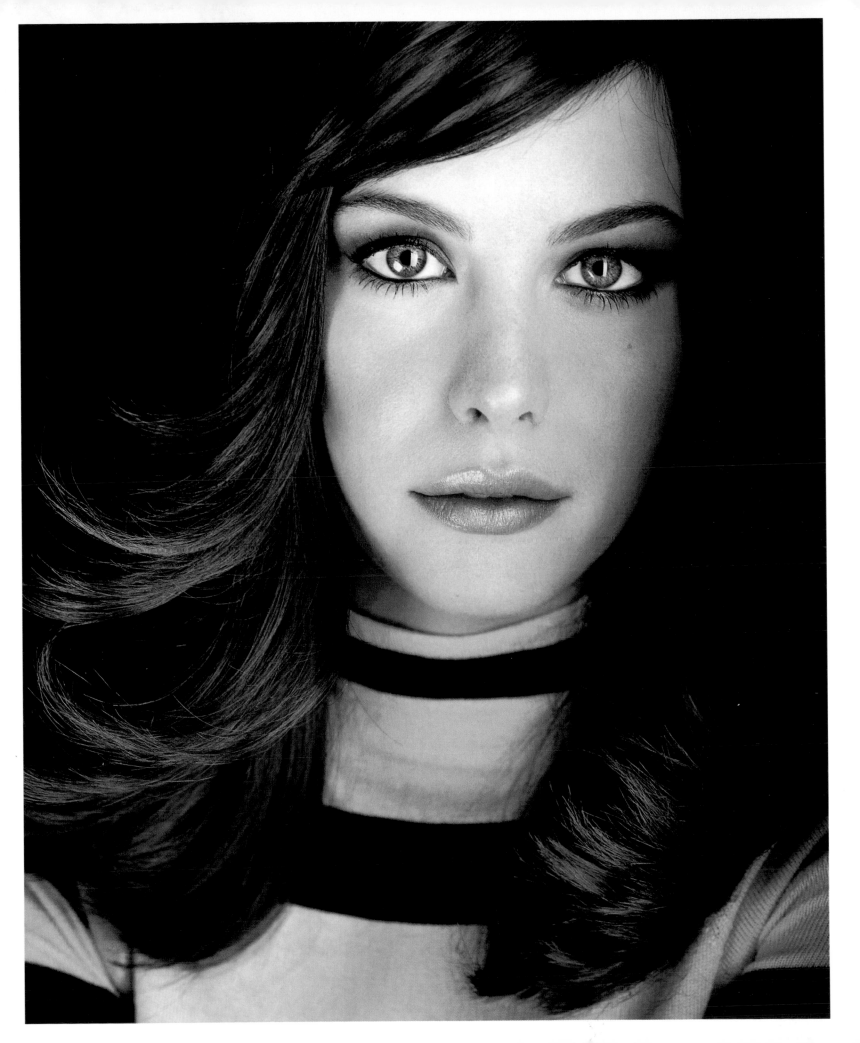

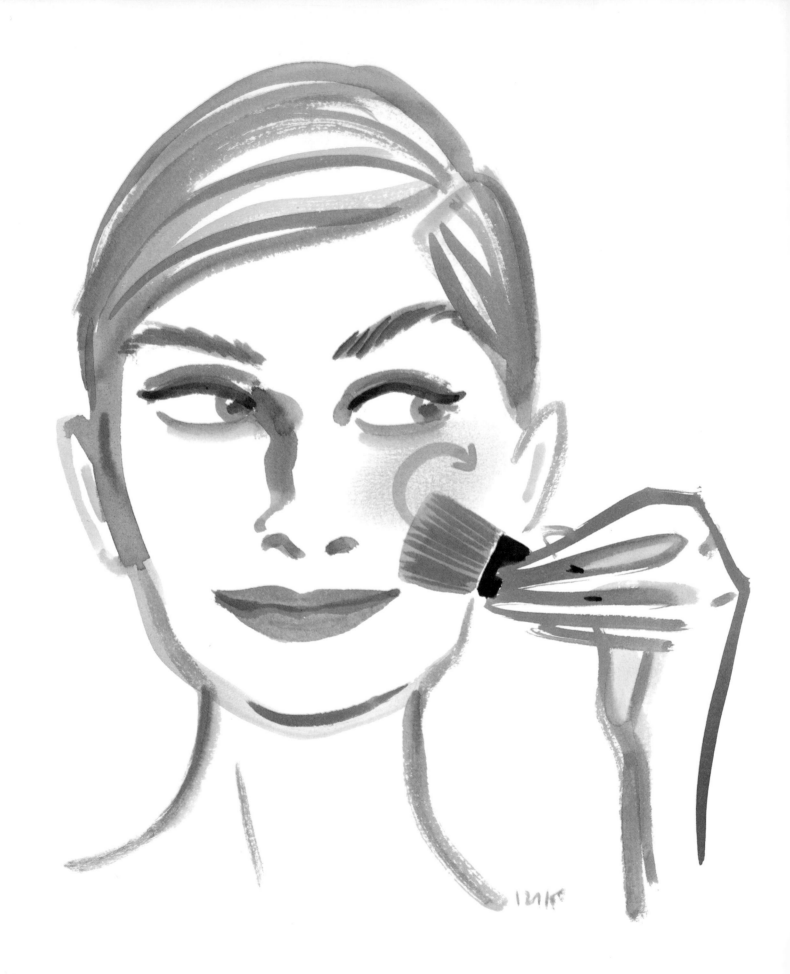

at once. (Doing so also protects the face products underneath, since it prevents you from moving and pushing everything around.) Deposit some color on the side of the brush, place the side against the apple of your cheek, and work the color around the surface. If you've never used your brush in this manner, it will take a little getting used to, but you'll come to prefer this technique.

Work in a round motion, but don't go too close to your nose. You can apply blush only to the apples of your cheeks, or you can work the blush toward your ear. Don't work the blush up along your temples. You want to embrace your cheekbones. If you've never done this, then put your fingers on the apples of your cheeks and follow your cheekbones. This will give you a sense of where they are and where your blush should go.

Blush for Your Face Shape

I've seen old beauty books that recommend a certain "shape" of blush depending on your face shape. I think this is a very old-fashioned way of thinking. Again, you want something natural-looking on your face, not something geometric. Obsessing over your face shape is a waste of time!

Apply your blush in a circular motion with the flat side of your brush

Laura Mercier is such a professional in the beauty business—

she's so revered. In Laura's hands, you look like yourself but

heightened. Glamorous but real.

    —Mariah Carey

Mariah Carey by Albert Watson

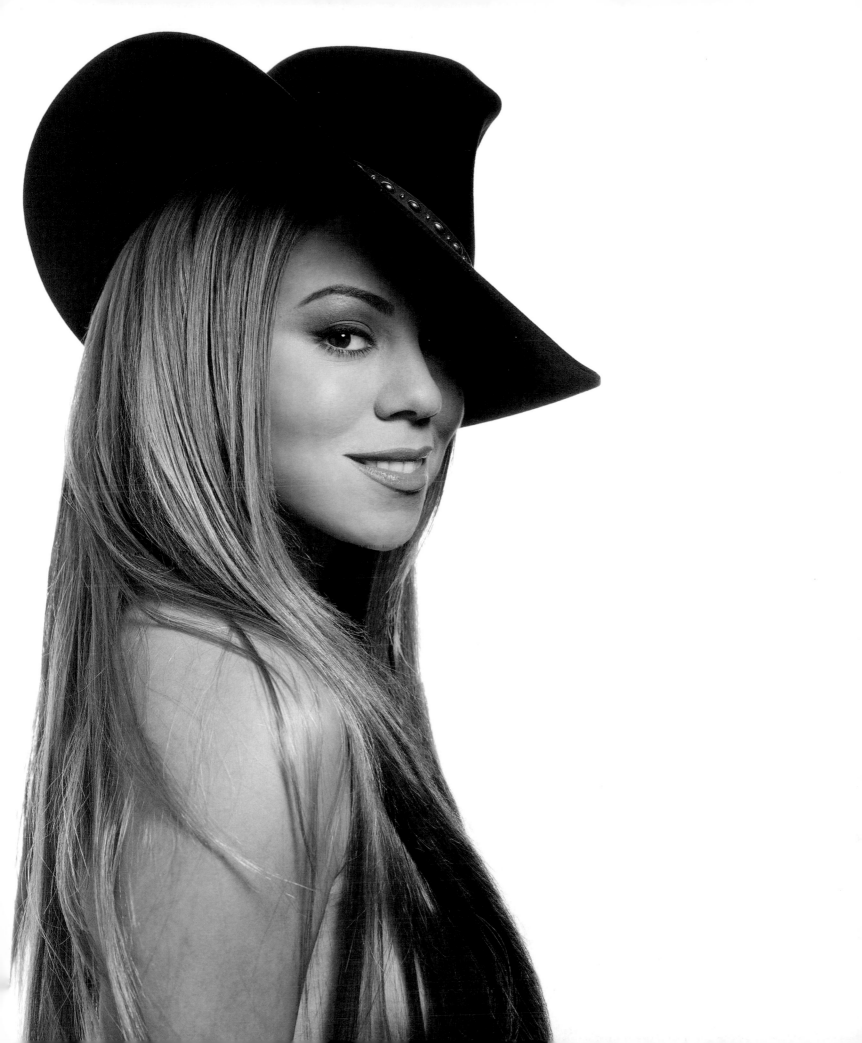

Blend Your Blush

If you have to blend your blush because you've applied too much and need to take some color away, then use a powdered puff. Prepare your puff by dipping it in translucent powder and patting against the back of your hand to remove any excess. Using the powdered side of the puff, blend where necessary. Don't use your fingers. It's best to use a soft, even surface with powdered blush.

You can blend away cream blush with your fingers if you applied too much. If the color is still very strong and you've simply used too much, you may need to remove the makeup and start over.

Counteract Dark Circles

If you have prominent circles under your eyes, blush can help distract from that area. When applying, do a full circle of color that embraces your cheekbones and goes right over part of the dark circle (which you've already covered with concealer). Again, blend well with your brush so it doesn't look like a very specific shape. This trick can also help you to balance out white circles under your eyes.

"Laura knows which parts of the face to play up and which parts to tone down—she has a real gift," says Isabella Rossellini. Photo by Michael Thompson.

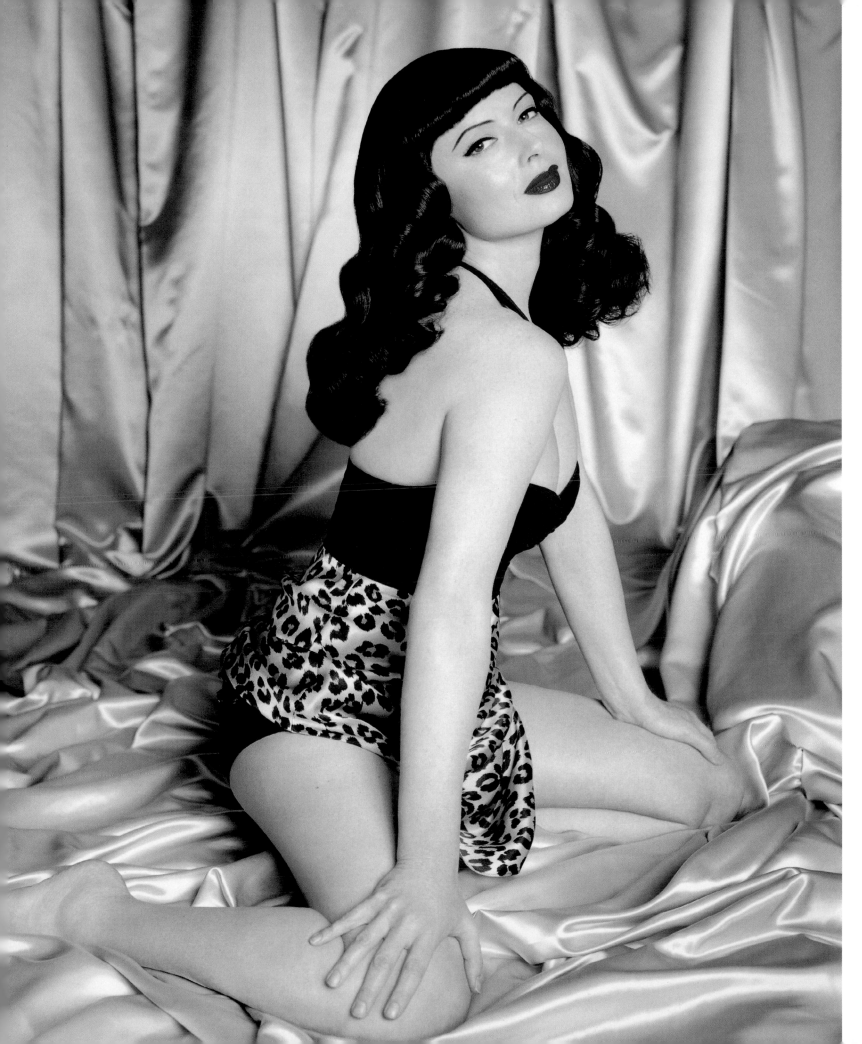

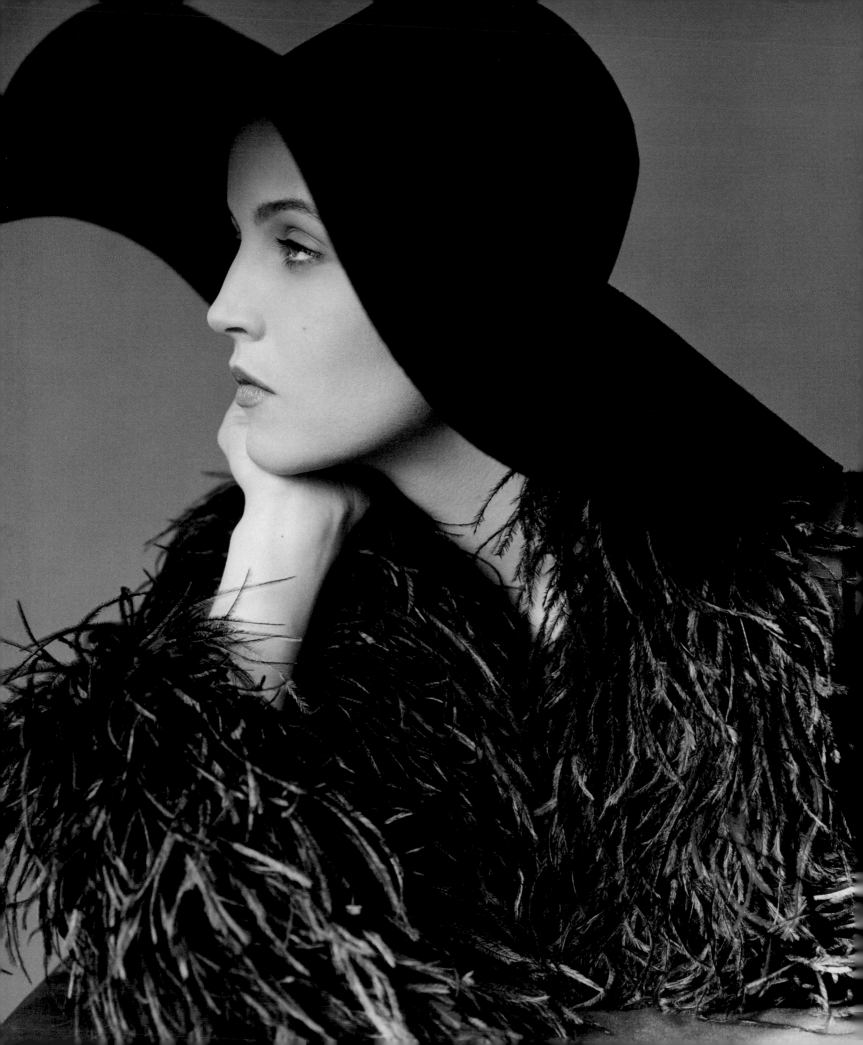

Balance is the key to a beautifully made-up face.

—Laura

Lisa Marie Presley, looking Garbo-esque, by Steven Meisel

Contouring with Blush

This is one of my big no-no's. You should never contour with blush because it's too colorful. Some women still apply blush to their temples, the tips of their chins, and their jawbones because it's the way they were taught and it's easier than having to use another product, but the result is a dated look that can be scary. Always use a specific contour product or matte bronzer, as we discussed in *The Flawless Face* chapter. The contouring will look more natural and fool the eye more successfully.

Liquid Blush

You can get a pretty, flushed look with this product, but it's not easy to use. It's almost impossible to blend because it dries so quickly. If your skin is very dry, tends to absorb products quickly, or both, you won't be able to blend it at all. If you'd like to try a liquid blush, I suggest applying it to bare skin. You can wear it alone or add product on top of it. Consider using a gel blush. It's in the same general family of products, but is easier to use.

A Kiss of Shimmer

The perfect finishing touch for your cheeks? A sexy, natural-looking glow. Shimmer sticks and blocks of shimmer powder are very popular products today, and they do the job beautifully by providing a translucent glow. They come in wonderful colors such as gold, silver, bronze, and rose-gold, and you can use them for daytime as long as they don't contain glitter. (If you're going to wear glitter at all, I'd save it for nighttime.) The idea behind shimmer is that it catches the light, so apply it right on the top center of the cheekbone where the light hits naturally. If you use the shimmer block, then apply it with a brush; if you use the shimmer stick, then dab it directly onto your finger and blend lightly over your cheeks so as not to disturb the blush underneath. Using your finger gives you more control. This is one of the few times you can break the cream-powder rule, so apply it directly on top of powder blush.

Don't apply translucent powder on top of shimmer products—you'll neutralize the shine.

Covering Acne on Your Cheeks

If you have pimples on your cheeks, I have a trick for covering them. If you wear foundation, apply it first and follow with a cream blush, or apply your cream blush alone. Next, take your camouflage and using the tip of your camouflage brush, erase the spots right on top of the cream color. Set with translucent powder and powder blush to even everything out. If you still see the blemishes, then retouch with a little camouflage and reset.

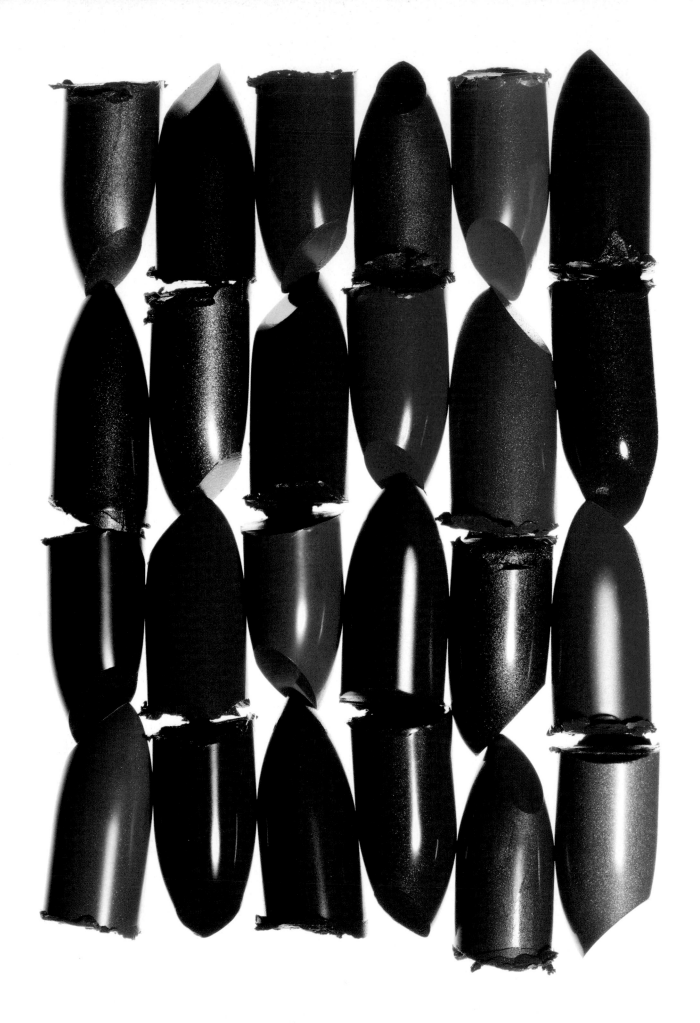

chapter seven lip service

If you're like most women, you love lip products. You probably have enough lipstick, lip gloss, or lip balm to last a lifetime, and I'll bet you've kept ones you haven't worn in years. "Maybe one day I'll need it," you think, contemplating the neglected tubes stored somewhere in your bedroom or bathroom.

If you're like me, you've gone through different lip phases where you're obsessed with one look. I've been through several, most notably my red period. For years, I wore nothing but matte red lipstick. No foundation. No eye makeup. Just crimson lips on a perfectly nude face. It reminded me of the glamour of old movies and was a way for me to feel more feminine and sexy. Plus, it was the eighties and I was living in Europe, where red lips were very much in fashion. When I moved to the United States, my look didn't work anymore because it felt too exotic. As the nineties dawned, red lipstick fell out of fashion and beiges and browns were all the rage. I looked terrible in those colors, so I had to find something else. Chocolate browns, especially those with a hint of red, worked well, as did chestnut lip liner, which I'm still addicted to today.

These days, anything goes when it comes to lips—matte hues, stains, glosses, tinted balms. I can't leave the house with naked lips, so I wear my beloved red lipstick, my favorite chestnut liner, raisin gloss, or plain lip balm depending on my mood and the situation. Maybe you have a signature shade, or you'd like to experiment with different lip looks. Whatever you need, I've got plenty of ideas for making your lips look as pretty as possible.

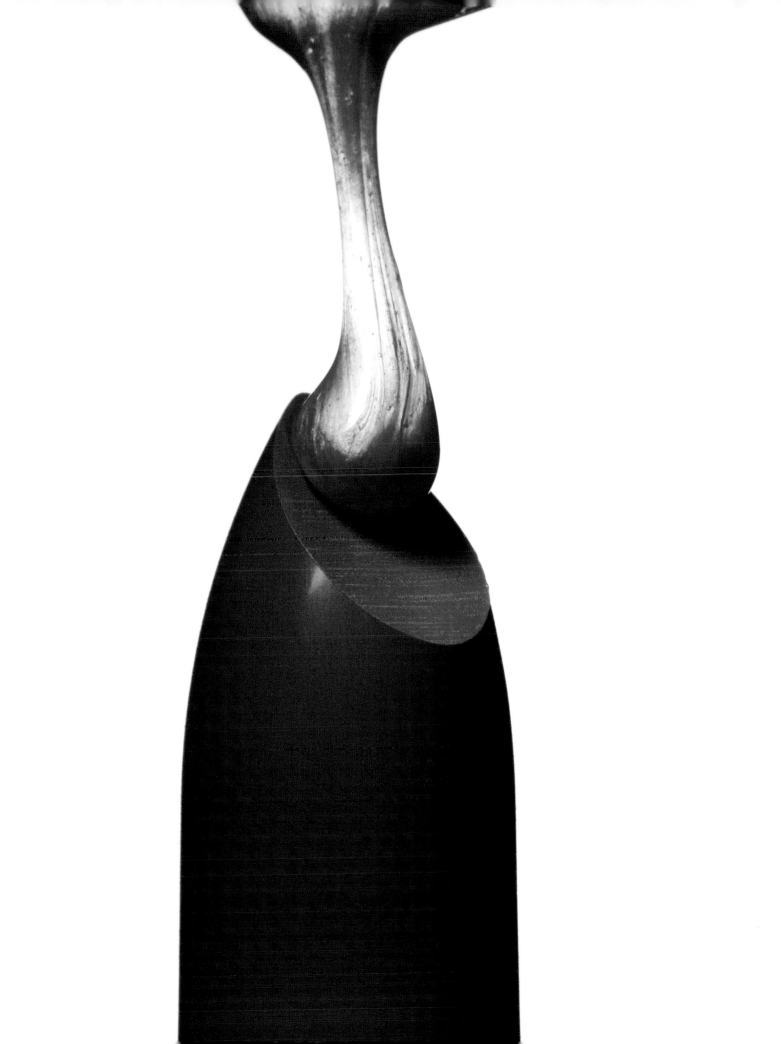

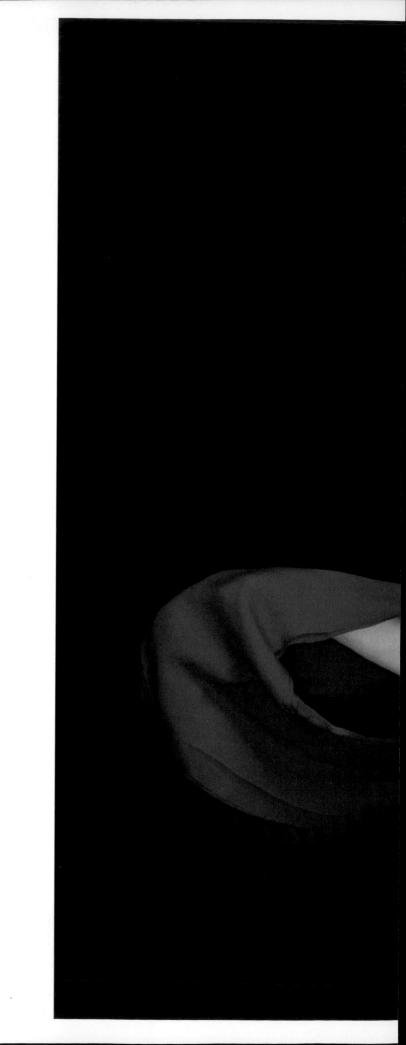

Laura Mercier is the Rembrandt of makeup artists.

—Madonna

Madonna by Patrick Demarchelier

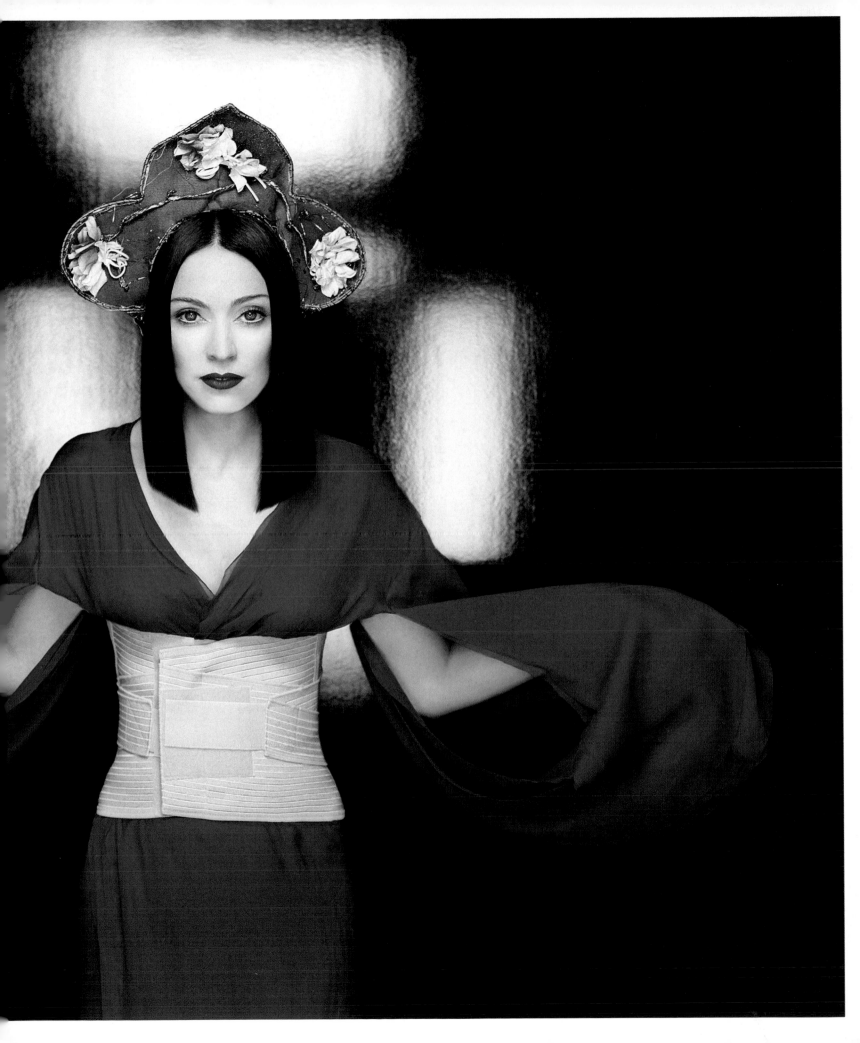

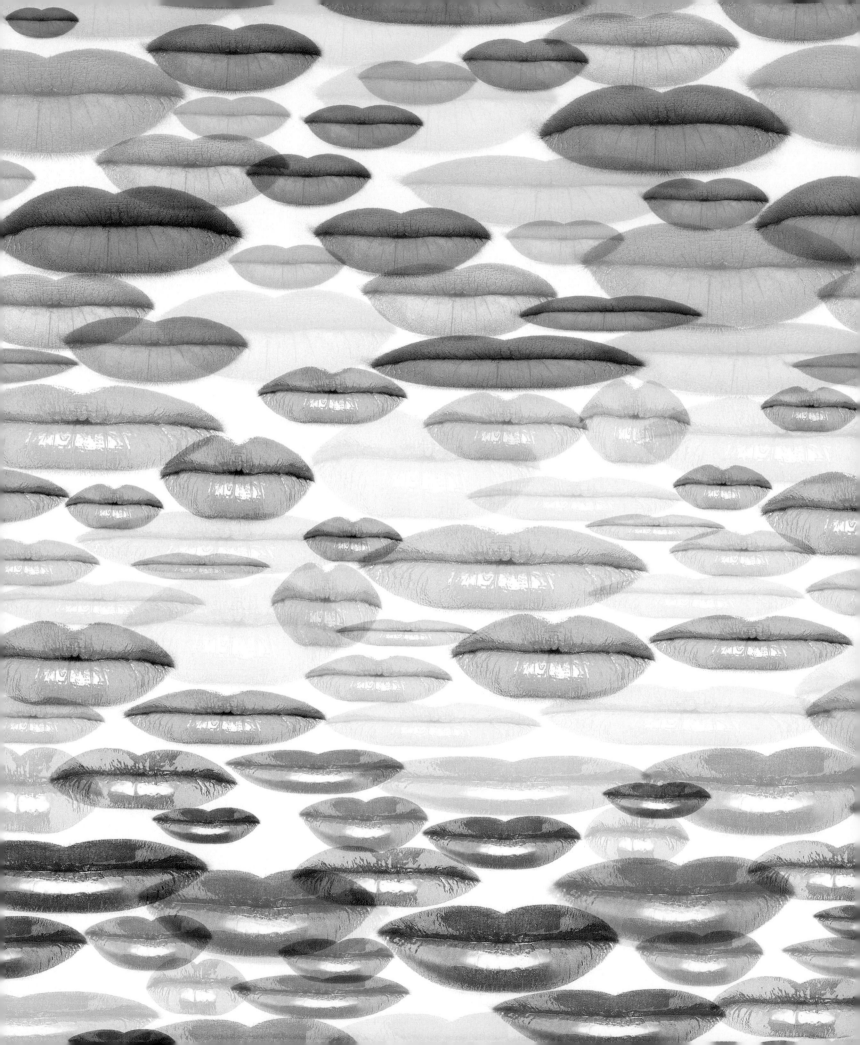

Treat Your Lips

Let's start with your lip care routine. This involves gently exfoliating your lips and treating them with a balm that both nourishes and moisturizes. Exfoliate as often as needed using a special lip scrub, a gentle face scrub, or even your toothbrush. Don't ever use anything harsh, like a loofah. The skin on your lips is much too delicate. I like to exfoliate my lips in the shower. Once I'm out, I cover them with a thick coat of balm. Give the lip balm time to sink in and do its job. Once you're ready to apply your makeup, wipe off the excess lip balm with some tissue. You don't want too much emolliency because your lipstick or lip gloss won't last as long.

You should also practice good lip habits such as drinking enough water. Your lips dry out quickly when you're dehydrated. Smoking is the worst habit for your lips because it stains, dehydrates, and cracks them.

The Right Shades for You

Once you understand the lipstick and gloss colors that are most flattering on you, you'll be able to create a variety of lip looks. Best of all, you won't waste money on colors that don't work. To begin, you need to know the lipstick or gloss tone that's right for your complexion. All shades can be divided into two families—warm tones and cool tones. The cool ones include anything with a hint of blue—mauves, fuchsias, milky pinks (imagine fuchsias mixed with white), purples, blue-reds, and berries, just to name a few. Warm tones have a hint of yellow or orange—browns, chestnuts, brown-pinks, beiges,

With a little experimentation, you'll find the right shade for you. Photo by Raymond Meier.

taupes, caramels, corals, and orange-reds. If your skin tends to be yellow or sallow, shades from the cool family will probably look best on you. Extreme warm tones tend to play up the yellowness of any complexion, so try them if your skin is on the pinkish side.

Experiment with different lipstick shades when you have no other makeup on your face. You'll be able to see which colors brighten your complexion and work best with your eyes and hair. You may find that you can wear warm and cool tones, or you may discover that one tonal family suits you best.

If you are always unsatisfied with your lipstick, mix two lipsticks or other lip products together to find the perfect color. Try mixing warm and cool tones. Don't be afraid to experiment.

What Is Your Lip Tone?

Another thing to consider when picking lipsticks or glosses is the natural color of your lips. A highly pigmented pout, be it pink, blue, or purple, will affect the shade of any lipstick or gloss you apply to your lips. This explains why a lipstick may look one way on you and another way on a friend or a model in a magazine. Keep this in mind when you sample lipstick on the back of your hand and wonder why it seems so different on your lips. It's because the undertones are completely different. Look for shades that complement or counteract your natural lip color.

Susan Sarandon by Sante D'Orazio

124

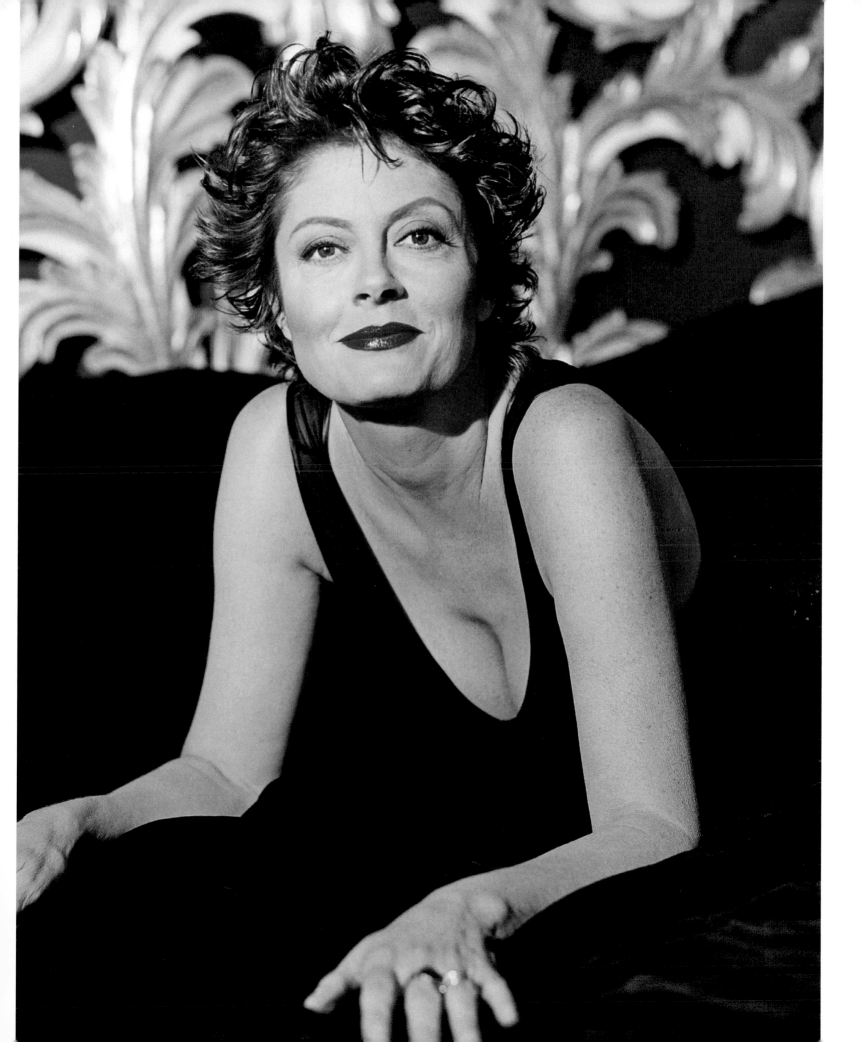

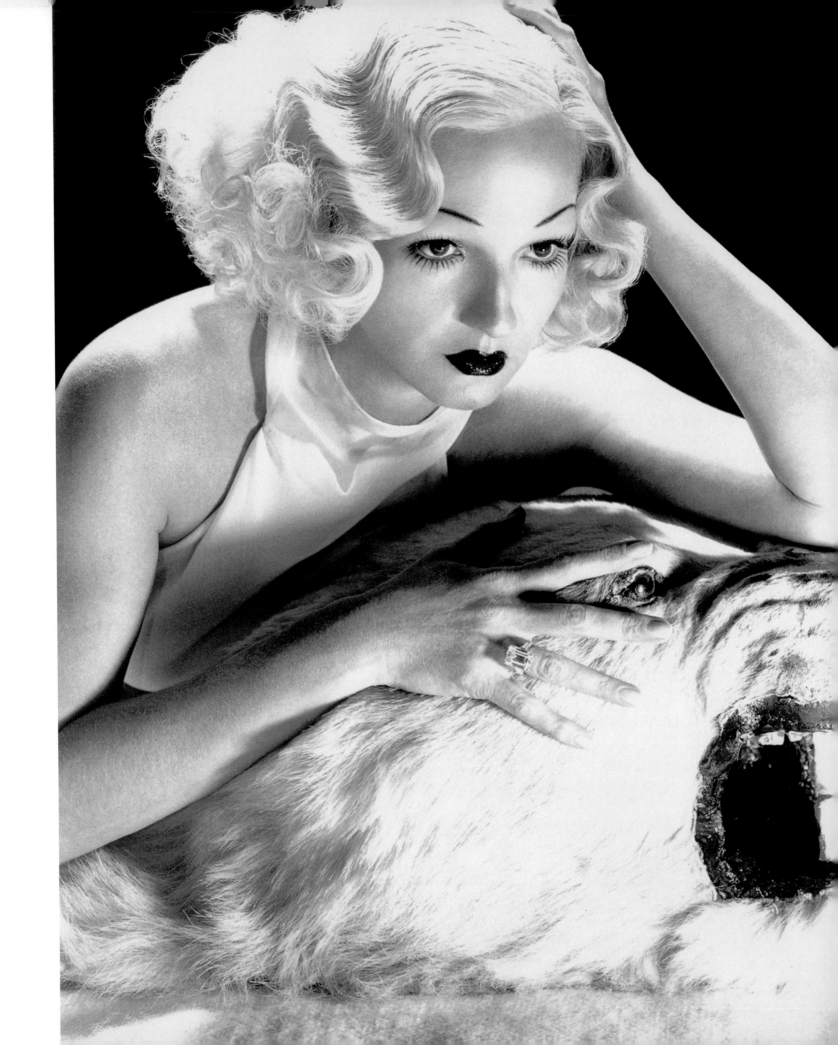

Never underestimate the power of dramatic lips.

—Laura

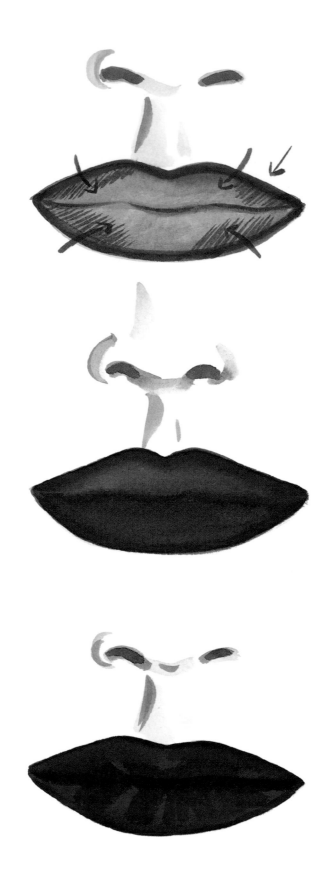

Getting Started

The next steps depend on the look you want and your needs. You can simply put on some gloss or sheer lipstick, or you can use a lip pencil to color your lips and cover it with lipstick or gloss. Since I'm sure you have these fundamentals down pat, I'm going to take you beyond the basics and teach you some advanced lip tricks.

Pencil Makes Perfect

Lip pencils are a great tool to use to make your lipstick last, correct any asymmetric proportions, provide definition, or make your pout larger. Make sure to chose a color that's a slightly enhanced version of your natural lip tone.

If you like the shape of your lips and just need a little definition, follow the outline of your mouth with the pencil. Next, color in the rest of the lips from the outside to the inside. It's like coloring inside the lines in a coloring book. You don't want to see a dark, obvious outline around lighter colored lips. Nothing's more old-fashioned, and it doesn't look elegant or sophisticated.

The Lip Canvas

For Serious Lipstick Work

Just as your face sometimes needs to be prepped before applying makeup, so do your lips. The tips and tricks that follow all require the same lip preparation, which I'm going to describe here. You need some camouflage, your lip pencil, translucent setting powder, and a powder puff. Using your finger, press a little camouflage into and around your lip line until it disappears into your skin. (Don't cover your lips entirely.) Dip your powder puff into a small amount of translucent powder and shake off the excess. The amount that remains is all you need. Press the puff very lightly over your lips. You want a surface that is dry, not dry-looking. Now your pout is prepped and ready for you to use your lip pencil as directed in the paragraphs that follow.

Get Bigger Lips (Naturally)

Almost everyone dreams of having sexier lips, but few people use their lip pencil correctly to achieve this look. Instead of drawing outside your entire lip line, just widen the middle of your top and bottom lips. (You may not need to do the top *and* bottom. Some people have naturally plumper bottom lips or vice versa.) Once you prepare your lips, raise the bow of your top lip by drawing slightly above it and reconnecting it at the middle on either side. Make the lower lip a little rounder at the center.

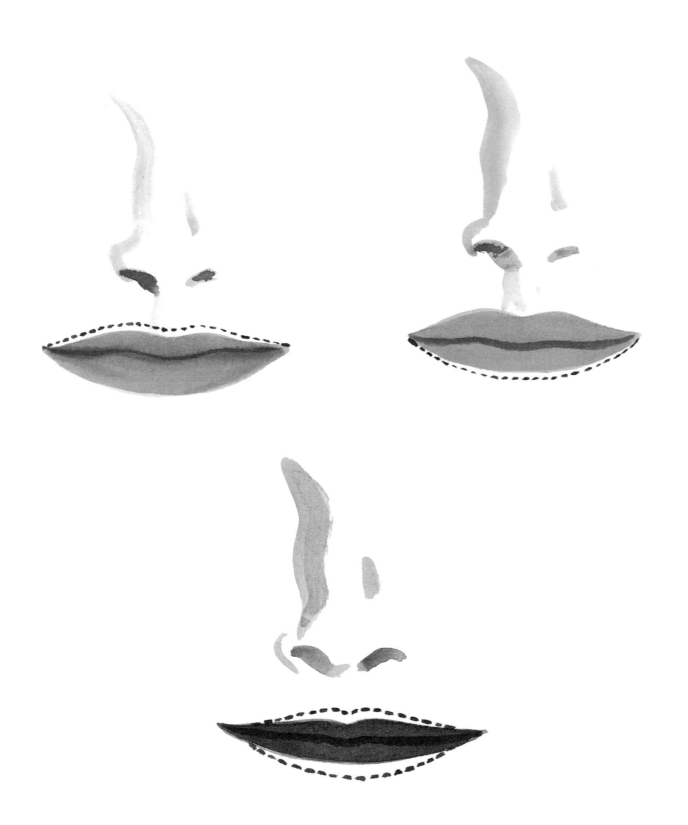

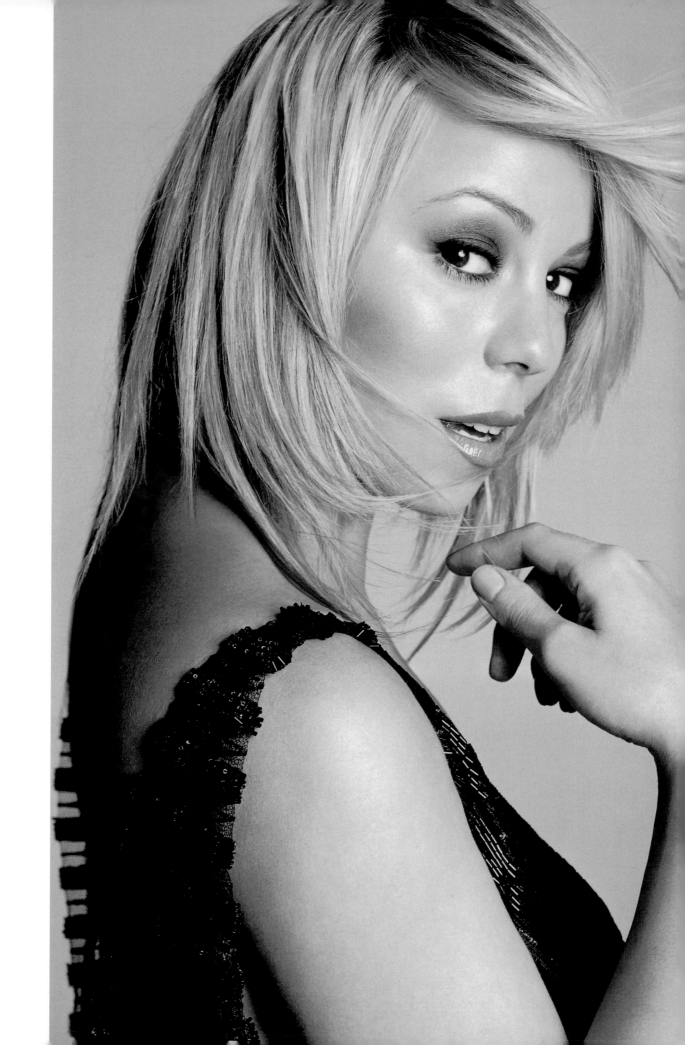

Laura knows how to make your facial features pop for the camera,

and my skin has never looked better than when she's done my

makeup. I don't know how she does it, but she understands what

kind of makeup is necessary for a really great photograph.

—Mariah Carey

Mariah Carey by Michael Thompson

This looks more natural and is an easier correction than going from corner to corner and drawing outside your entire mouth. The exception to this rule is if you have very thin lips. In this case, you can draw outside the entire lip line to enhance its appearance. Don't forget to fill in the space between your natural lip line and the correction.

If your lips are asymmetric, then you can use a pencil to correct them. Again, make sure your lips are prepped correctly. This will help you draw in the shape more beautifully and help the color last longer.

Make Your Lipstick Last

There are long-wearing lipsticks on the market today that can last for hours, but they tend to dry out your lips, so you're sacrificing comfort for practicality. Instead, prep your lips as described in The Lip Canvas section. The camouflage and powder set the lip liner and the lip liner serves as an anchor for your lipstick or gloss.

You can take it one step further and create a matte finish for your lipstick. After you've powdered over your lined lips, apply a coat of lipstick. Take one layer of tissue and press it against your lips to blot away any excess oils. (Lipstick tends to fade because your lips absorb the oil in the lipstick's formula for hydration. This technique helps your lipstick last longer since it removes some of the oils.) Take a second layer of tissue, put it over your lips, and powder with a puff *over* the tissue. This allows a fine layer of powder through and helps you avoid applying too much powder. It also protects your puff at the same time. If you desire, you can apply a second coat of lipstick for a creamier look, but avoid the contours of your mouth so the lipstick lasts longer.

Kate Moss by Steven Meisel

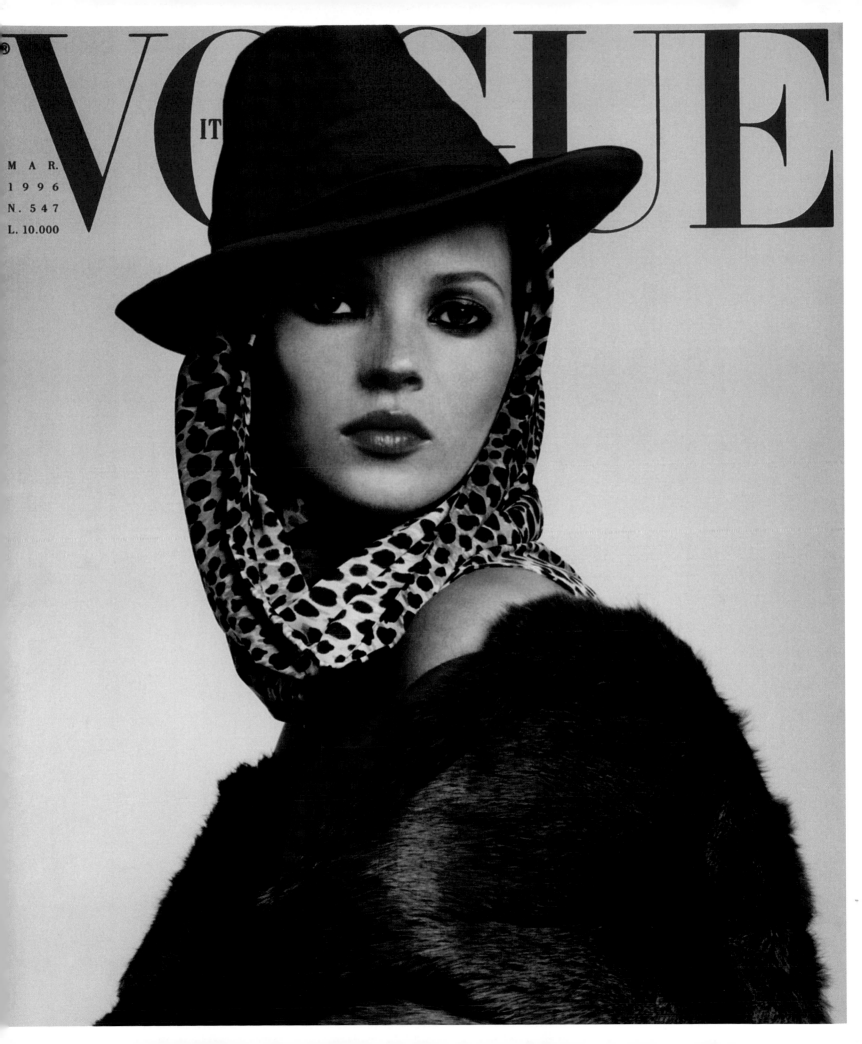

VOGUE

IT

MAR.
1996
N. 547
L. 10.000

Obviously, lots and lots of makeup go into magazine photo sessions, even

if it's a so-called "natural" look—and Laura has the gift of applying that

makeup perfectly. She's a painter who uses women's faces as her

canvas—and being a woman, she brings out the best of feminine beauty.

　　—Julianne Moore

Julianne Moore by Michael Thompson

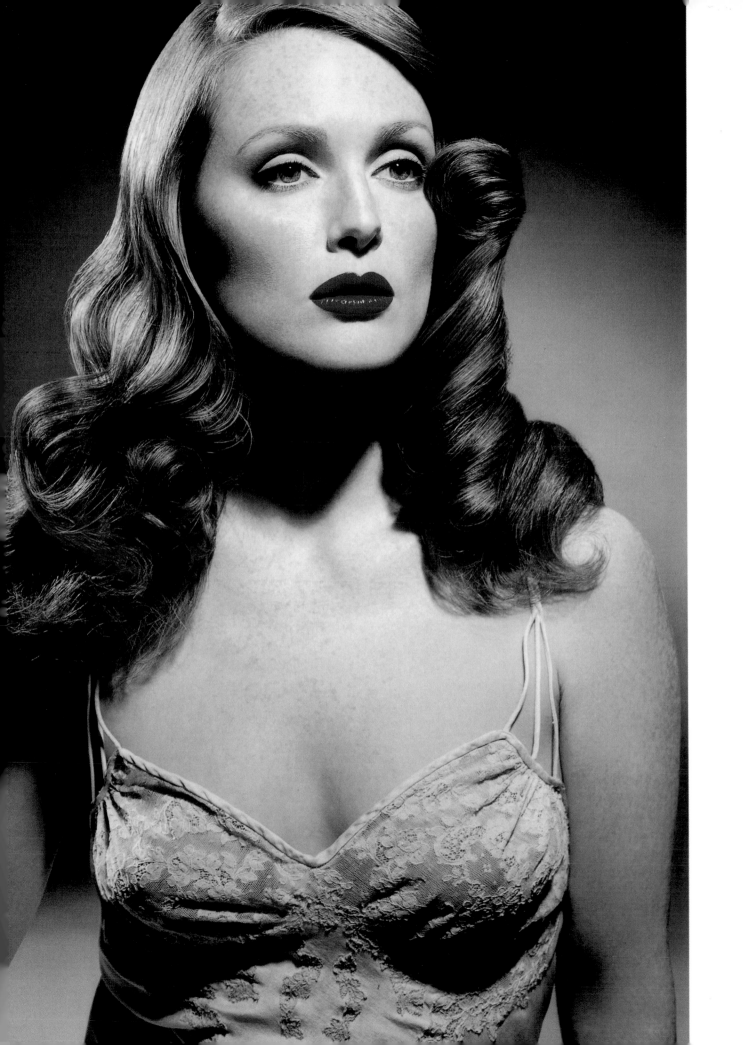

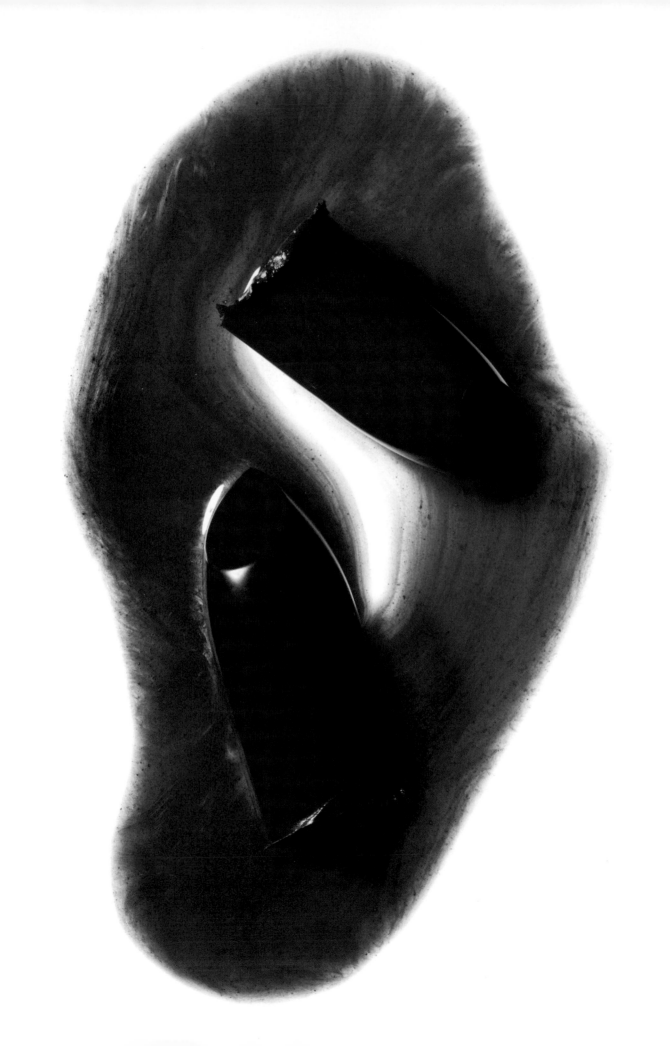

Prevent Bleeding and Feathering

Nothing's worse than lipstick or lip gloss that migrates beyond your lip line. Sometimes it occurs because your lips and the surrounding skin get drier and more wrinkly with age; sometimes the formula of the lipstick is very oily for intense hydration. Light, liquidy lip glosses, for example, have a tendency to travel. The thicker and/or drier the formula, the more likely it will stay put.

If you want to prevent your lipstick from bleeding or feathering, follow the previous steps for making your lipstick last because it will certainly help keep your lipstick in place. If you use lip gloss, follow The Lip Canvas prep, and apply gloss to only the center of your mouth. Make sure the gloss doesn't hit your lip line to achieve the sexy shine of gloss; the camouflage, powder, and lip liner provide a barrier.

Many women think they can't wear gloss as they get older, but this trick should help. Lip gloss is great for older lips because it makes lips look plumper by catching the light. If you wear a little as a point of light, you'll get the benefits of gloss without any mess.

> **beauty secret >** Matte lipsticks work better in certain climates than others. If you live somewhere humid, you're in luck because your lips are plumped by the moisture in the air. If you live somewhere arid like Arizona, matte lipstick probably isn't the best choice for you. Even with balm, your lips are going to be dry so try a moisturizing, creamy lipstick formula instead.

My Timeless Lip Looks

Red Lips

I mentioned my love affair with red lipstick earlier in this chapter. Many women are afraid to wear red because it's such a statement, or they worry that their lips are too small to pull off such a strong color. If you've never worn red, then you should give it a try. Red is not for everyone, but I know many women who would look heavenly wearing it for specific occasions and with the right look. It can boost your confidence and personality in unexpected ways. As to the size of your lips, it's true that dark colors make petite pouts look even smaller, but I know plenty of women in this category who wear red lipstick so much so that it has become their signature. If your lips are on the small side, keep your red light and bright and keep the rest of your makeup minimal.

If you do experiment with red, don't reserve it for a soiree or a big night out. I love red lips with casual clothes. To me, the less dressed up you are and the less makeup you are wearing, the more modern your red lips will look. Another way to keep the look modern is to not line your lips and apply the lipstick lightly, as a stain.

Bitten Lips

The fashion photographer Steven Meisel and I have worked together often throughout the years, and he coined bitten lips as a term. He would ask me to make the models' mouths look pretty and natural as if they had bitten their lips and done

Madonna, in the striking combination of red lips and fuchsia-accented eyes. Photo by Patrick Demarchelier.

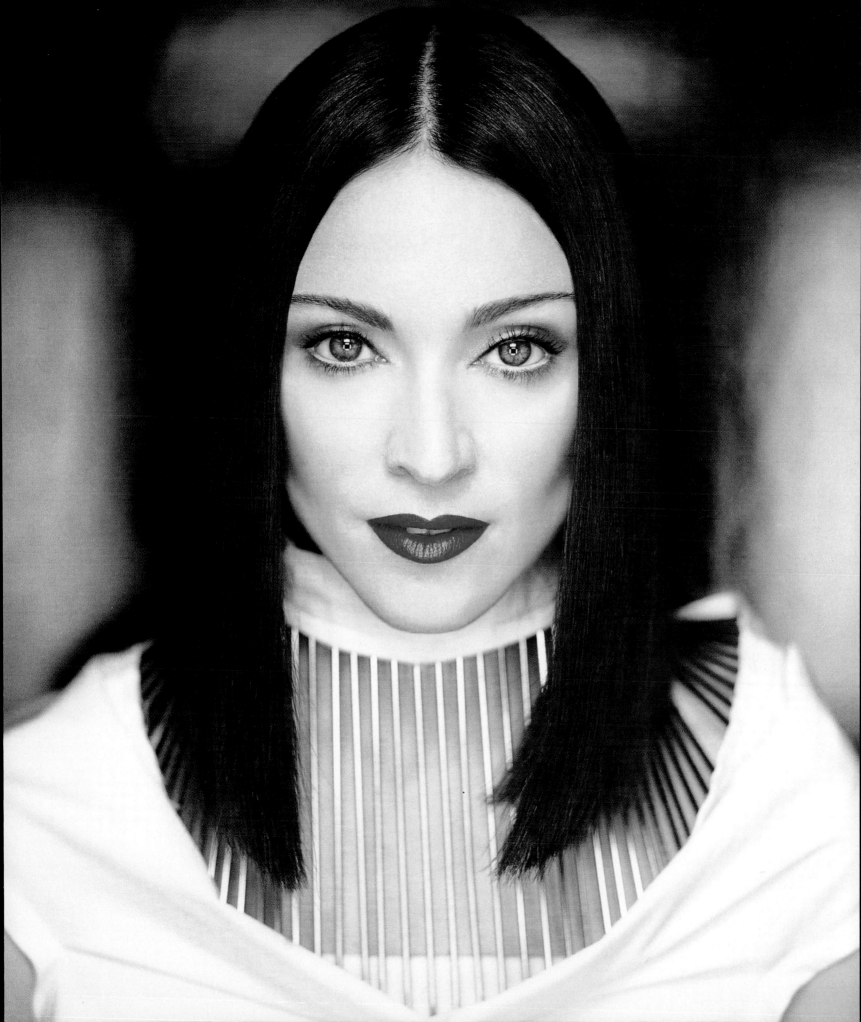

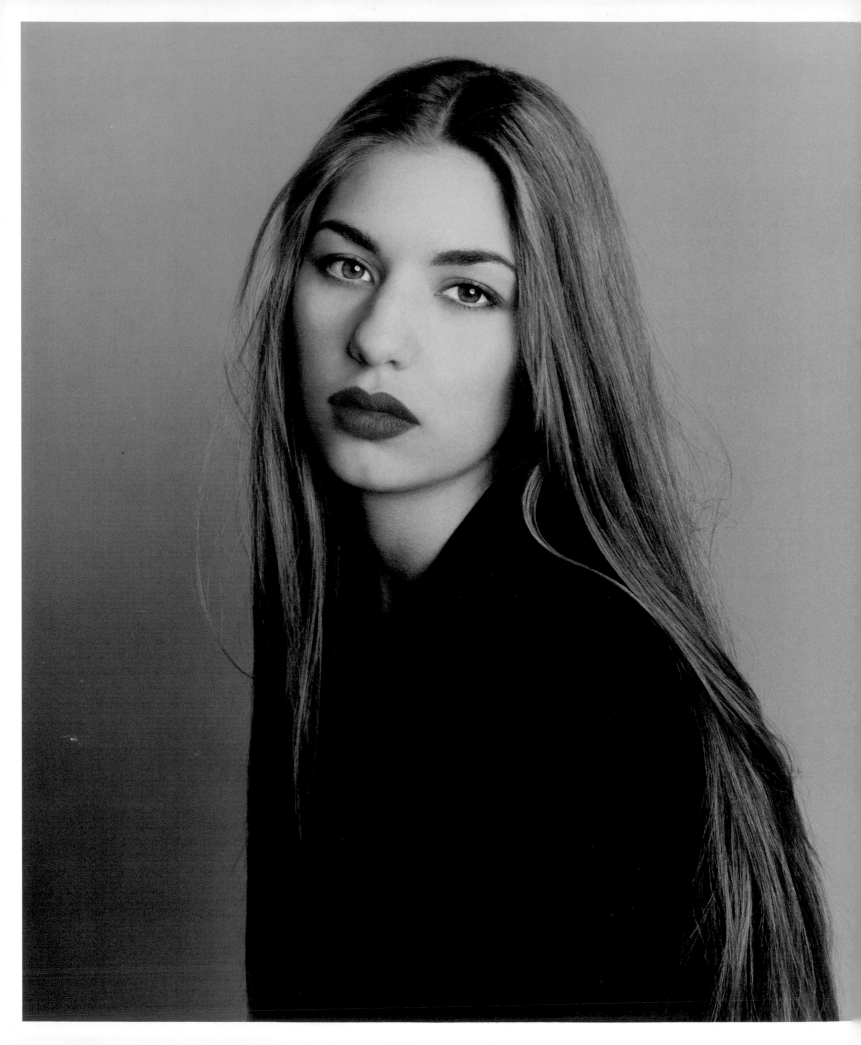

nothing else. So I would dab on a brownish-red color to mimic that look. The idea was to lightly stain the lips with lipstick. You can give yourself "bitten lips" or you can make the look more intense—think of your lips after you've had some red wine or a cherry popsicle.

This trick is very easy to do. Just rub or dab your finger over your lipstick and apply by pushing the product onto your naked lips. It could be any color—corals, pinks, reds, burgundies—but the effect you're going for is watercolor. This is great for women who don't want to wear traditional lipstick but want something other than gloss. It's also a safe way to wear red as mentioned before or any darker colors without it being so obvious. It's a much softer, more natural-looking approach.

Naturally Sexy Lips

One of my favorite looks for many of my celebrity clients and me is chestnut liner blended lightly over the entire lip and softened with your finger. (You're not doing any type of correction, nor are you penciling in the color with a heavy hand.) For the final step, dot some lip balm over your mouth. If chestnut liner is too dark for you, then try a lighter natural shade. The final effect doesn't look like you're wearing any makeup, but it gives you a very pretty, pouty look that's all your own.

Sofia Coppola by Steven Meisel

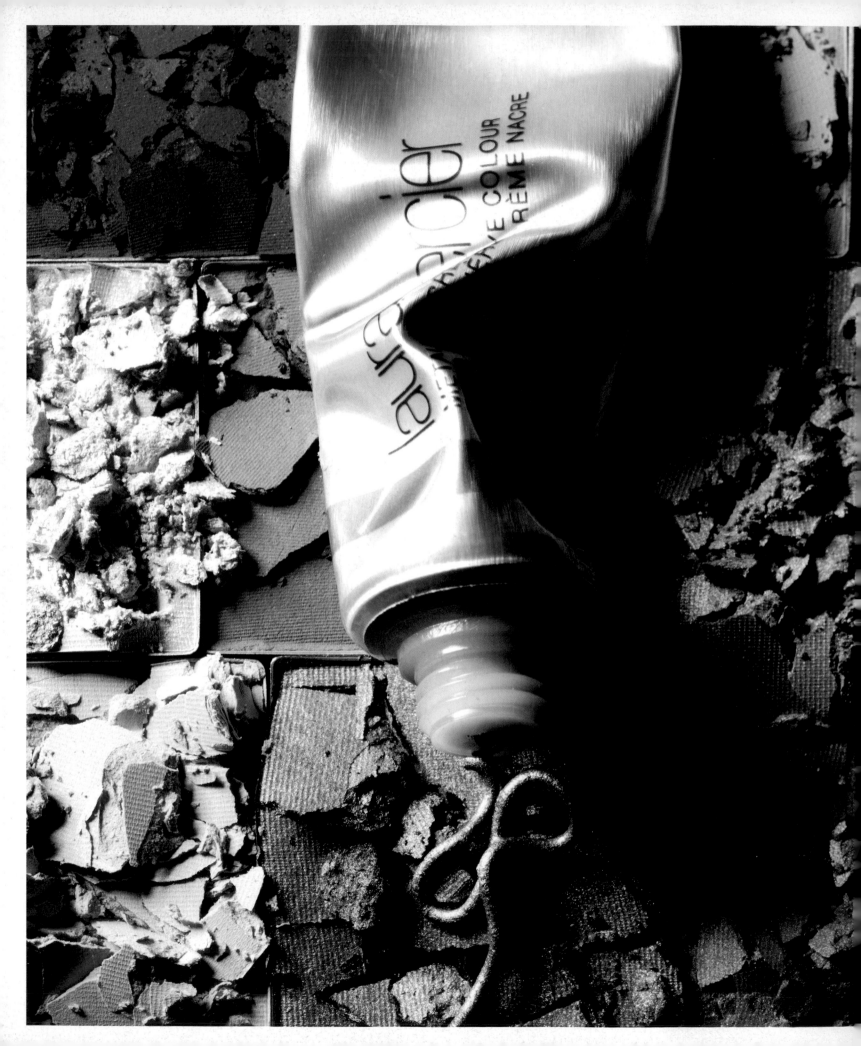

chapter eight bright eyes

With the exception of a signature lip color, eye makeup is the best way to show your personality via cosmetics. It's certainly the best way to display your creativity. Your eyes are your most flirtatious feature, and they're the one place on your face where almost anything goes in terms of color. Whether you opt for lush eyelashes, graphic eyebrows, or beautiful washes of shadow on your eyelids, your eye makeup says so much about you and your style.

At the same time, doing your eye makeup can be the trickiest part of your beauty routine. One of the most frequent requests at Laura Mercier counters is: "Show me what to do with my eyes." I'll give you plenty of options in this chapter and help you realize that mastering eyeliner and shadow is within reach. Perhaps applying eye makeup is already your forte. If that's the case, read on for ways to update your look, learn new techniques, and help your makeup last longer.

What Is Your Eye Shape?

I've already mentioned that face shape doesn't matter enough for you to obsess over, so does your eye shape really make a difference? It makes a huge difference! Understanding you eyes' shape will help you realize what looks work for you and, just as important, the looks that don't—which simplifies your eye makeup options because you'll know how to emphasize and draw attention to your eyes. The information that follows is meant to be a general guide, not a strict set of rules, so don't feel constricted by them. Also, your eyes may fit into more than one category, so keep that in mind when determining your course of action.

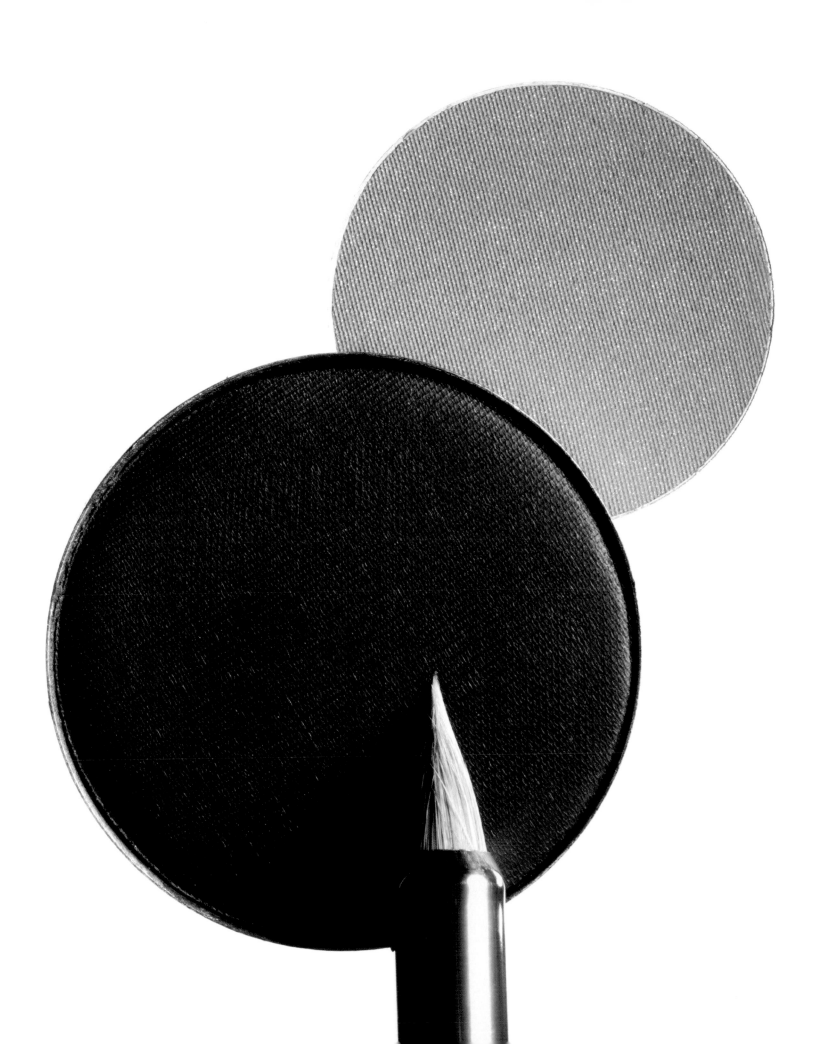

The Most Common Eye Shapes

Close Set Eyes

Apply a light-colored shadow closest to your nose and gradually darken the color horizontally toward the temple to visually add space between your eyes. If you don't want to use a lot of eye makeup, smudge a medium- to dark-intensity matte shadow or pencil at the outer corners. Another simple trick is to use medium or dark liner along the upper lash line and elongate the line at the outer corner.

Note: Lining around your entire eye and wearing dark colors on the inner half of your lids will make your eyes look as if they are closer together. When lining your eyes, start the liner away from the inner corners.

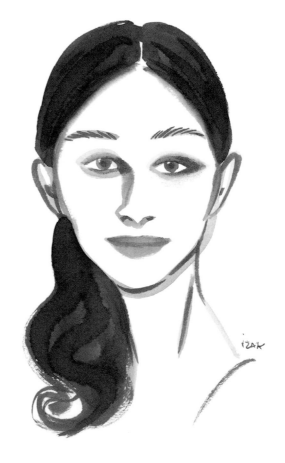

Wide Set Eyes

Apply a medium-intensity matte shadow on the inner half of your lids toward the nose and lighter shadow on the outer half to make it seem as if your eyes are closer together. You can also emphasize the crease with a medium-intensity shade, and blend the crease color toward the nose. Or you can line the entire eye. Just make sure to focus the intensity right at the beginning of the inner corner.

Note: Dark shadows on the outer corners and any winged eyeliner effects will emphasize the wide set nature of your eyes and make them look as if they are even further apart. Don't wear shimmer on the inner corners because it will attract the light and open the area, which is the opposite of what you want to try to do.

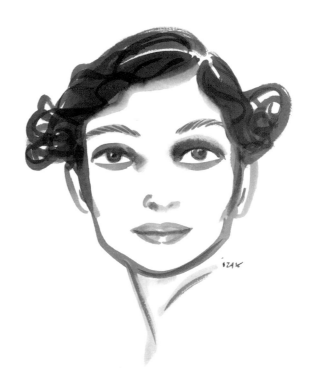

beauty secret > You've probably seen eyeliners that come in beige, icy blue, or white. These are used on the fleshy part of your lower lash line to make eyes look as if they are larger or more awake. It's a great trick for small eyes, deep set eyes, or both. These pencil colors open the eye by giving the illusion of pushing back the lash line. Don't use a pencil that's too chalky colored because it can look too obvious and ruin the illusion. I prefer a very soft baby-blue or off-white liner.

Deep Set Eyes

You want light and/or shimmery color on the lids from the lash line to the crease to the brow bone to pull the eyes forward. You can also line along the middle of the upper and lower lashes, avoiding the inner and outer corners. (You can line a bit below the lower lash line to make the eye seem larger than it is.) By not closing or connecting the eyeliner you're not shrinking the eye. You also can use medium to dark shadow or liner at the outer corners to pull the eyes out or simply define the upper lash line at the base of the lashes.

Note: Avoid wearing dark eye shadow on your lids and lining around your entire eye.

Downcast Eyes

Working at the outer corners, bring the shape up and in at a right angle using medium- or dark-intensity matte shadow. (Make sure to

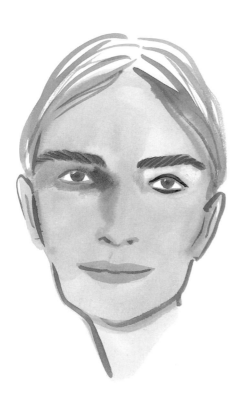

Flirty lashes and glossy lips by Marc Hispard

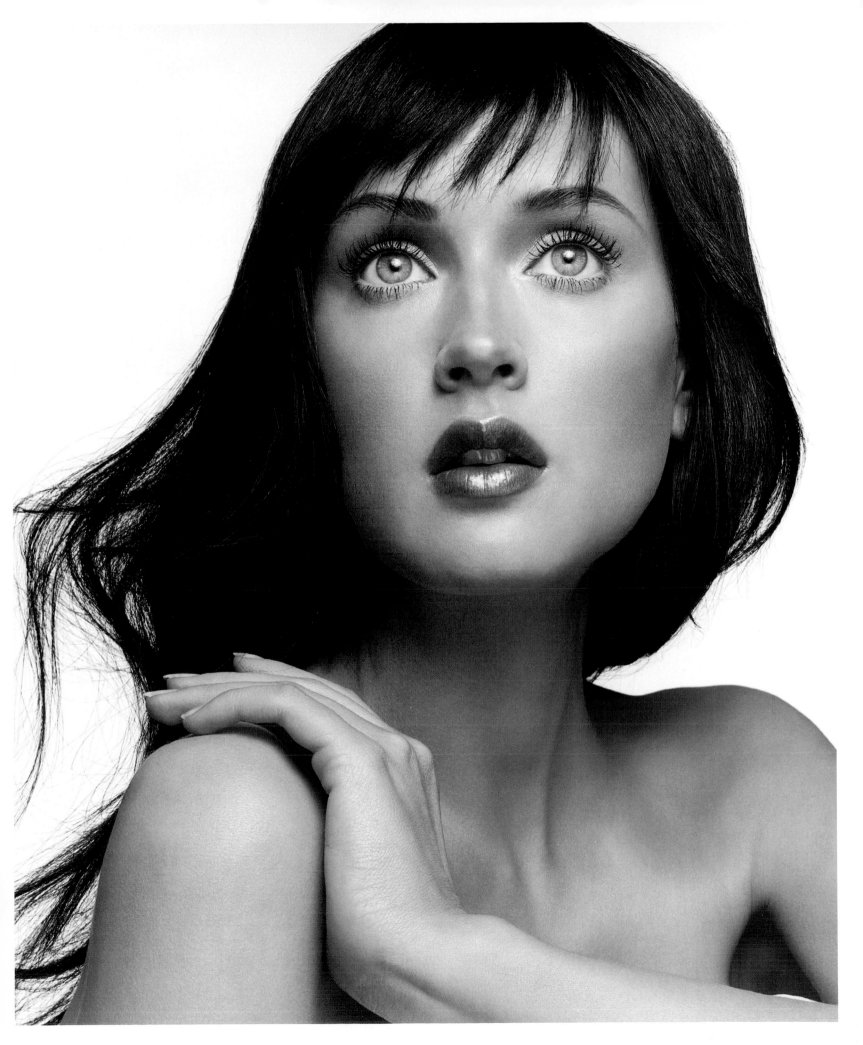

One of the wonderful things about

working with Laura is her vitality.

    —Julia Roberts

Julia Roberts by Michael Thompson

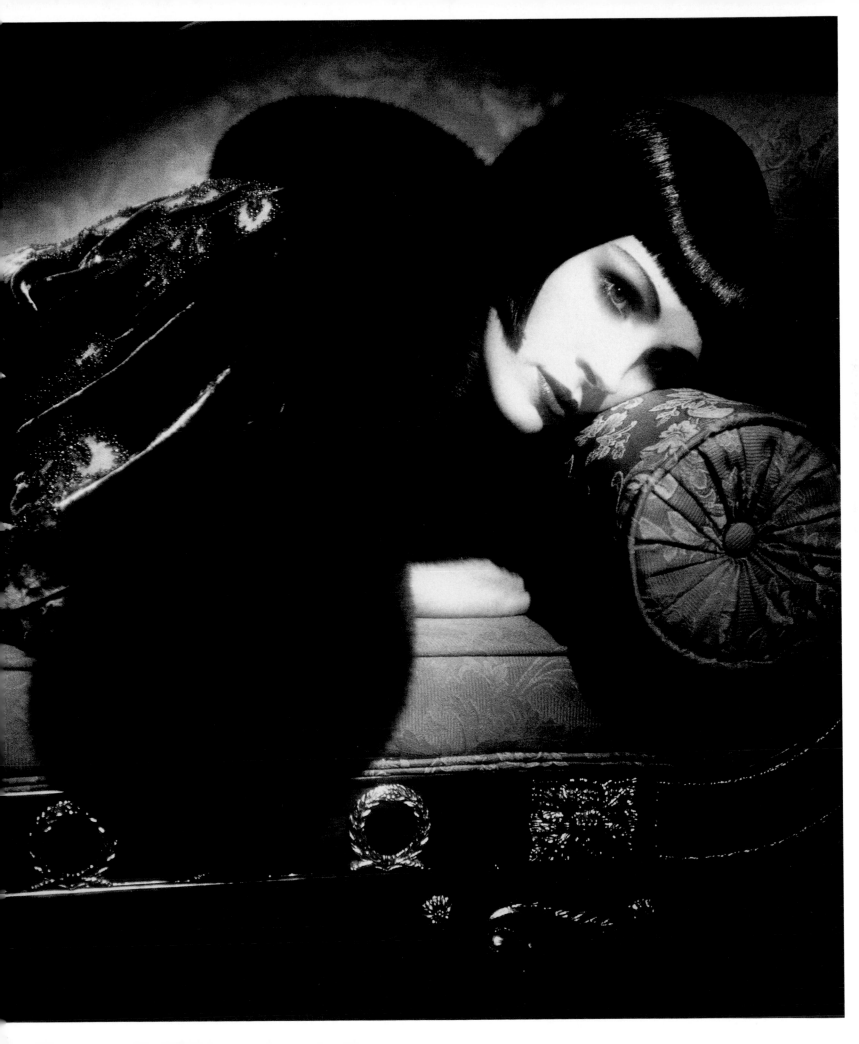

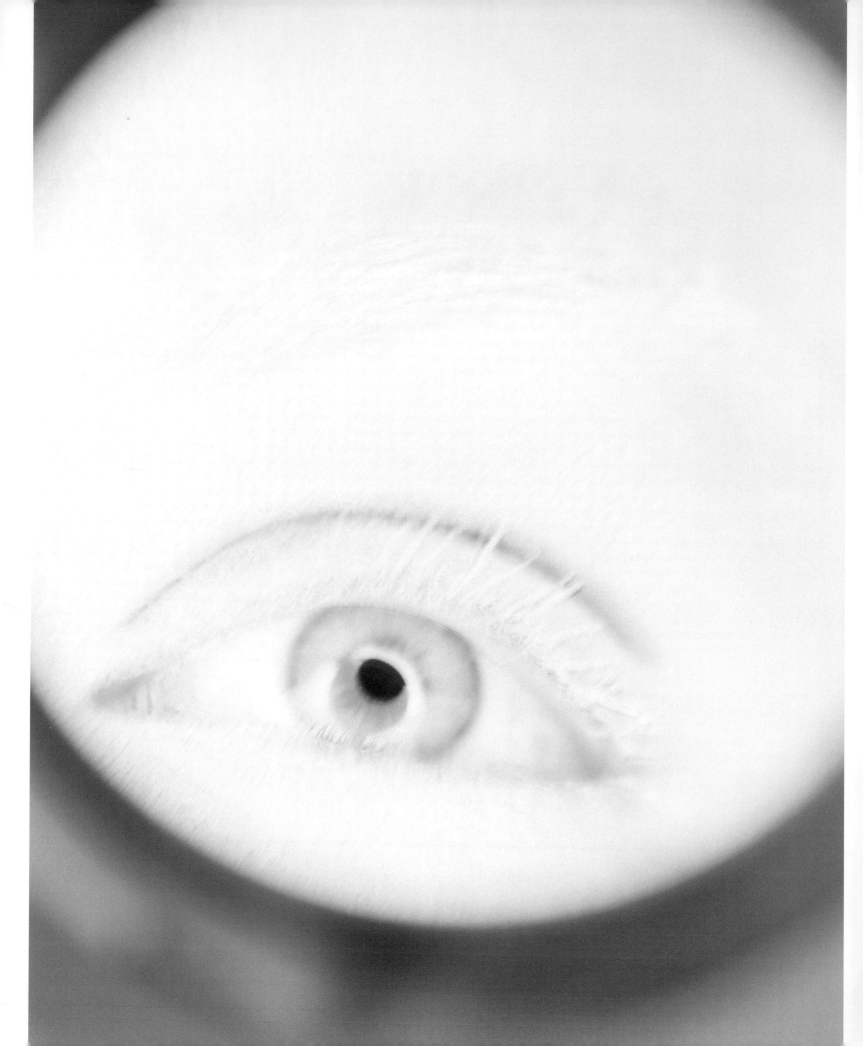

smudge the angle; you don't want a defined shape.) Don't follow the natural downward shape of the eye all the way. You want a soft upward motion. You can line the upper lid, but make it heavier at the end by smudging your pencil up a bit, rather than following the lash line down. Attract attention to the upper lid, not the downward corner.

Note: Don't line underneath the eyes.

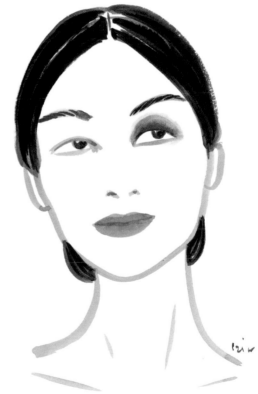

Creaseless Lids

Use shadow that goes from dark or medium matte to light gradually, from the lash line to the brow. You can also do color that graduates from light on the inner corners to dark or medium on the outer corners (also great for close set eyes). You can line around the entire eye as long as your eyes aren't close set or downcast.

Note: Don't try to create a crease.

White on white by Raymond Meier

Heavy Lids

Use a medium matte shadow from the lash line to the crease. If you have a little lid visible above the lash line, you can use a pale shimmery shadow to highlight that area. You can line your eyes right at the lash line and/or define your lash line at the roots (see note below) with cake or liquid liner.

Note: If you want to lift the eyes, don't do too much underneath with eyeliner. Keep it simple or don't do anything at all.

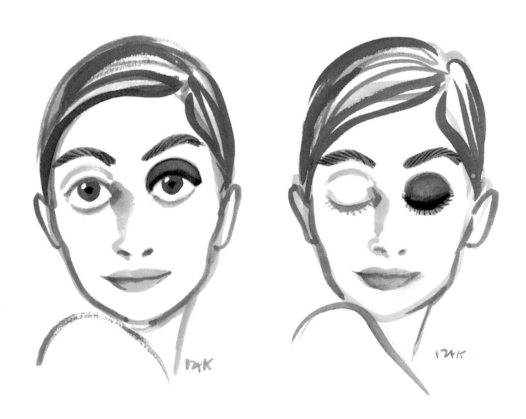

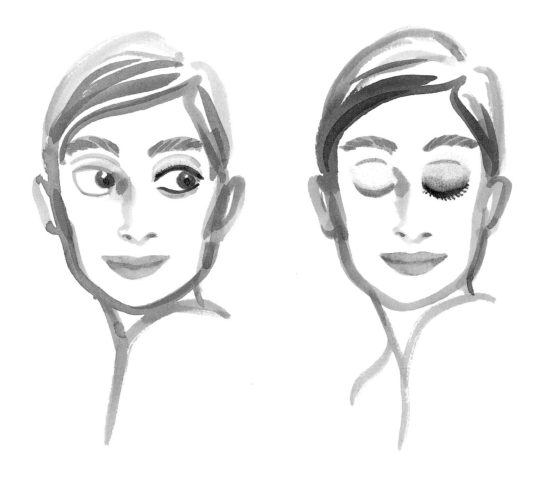

Prominent Eyes/Round Eyes

This eye type, by definition, has a lot of eyelid. You can use shadow and liner to visually diminish the size of the lid. Try a dark or medium matte shadow from the lash line to the start of the crease or use shadow that graduates from dark to medium, from the lash line to the crease. Use a flesh-colored or light shadow from the crease up. You also can use strong, thick eyeliner above the eye, or you can line around the entire eye (unless they are downcast or close set).

Note: Light and/or shimmery shadow on the eyelid will emphasize the eyelid by catching the light there and making it more prominent. Don't darken the crease.

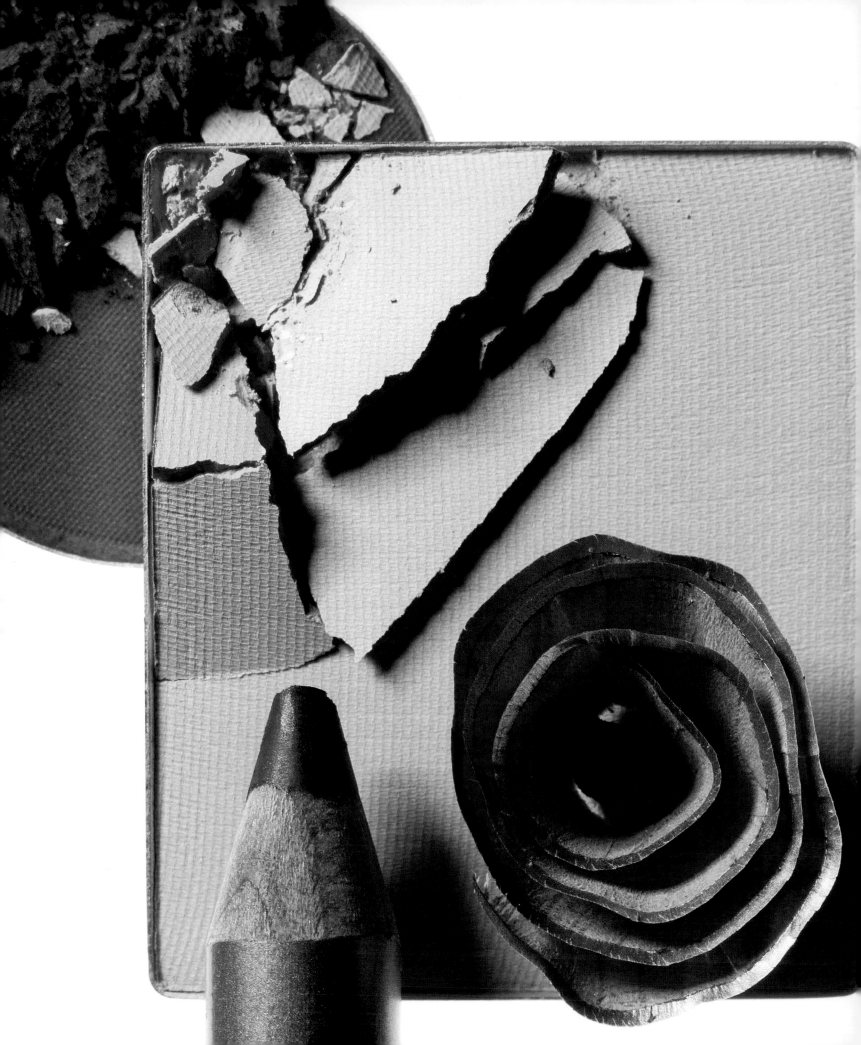

Don't Be Afraid of Color

The majority of women stick to neutrals when it comes to their eye makeup, but you should give color a chance from time to time. It's a great mood enhancer. I know psychiatrists sometimes tell their patients to stop wearing black because it has a way of drowning you emotionally and sapping your energy. Think about why you reach for a certain red blouse or blue sweater. It might seem arbitrary, but perhaps your psyche needs the calming effects of a specific hue or the energizing effects of a particular shade. Consider that the next time thoughts of violet eyeshadow or forest green liner pop up in your mind. Maybe you should trust yourself and give them a try. Follow your instincts! There is always a way to wear color—whether light, pale, or muted—that won't be intimidating.

Intensify Your Eye Color

There are simple ways to make your natural eye color really dazzle. As you probably know, certain colors complement and enhance other colors. The same theory works with eye makeup and your iris (the colored part of your eye). You can make your blues bluer, greens greener, and so on. I've found that the following basic color combinations work the best:

Your eye makeup says so much

about you and your style.

    —Laura

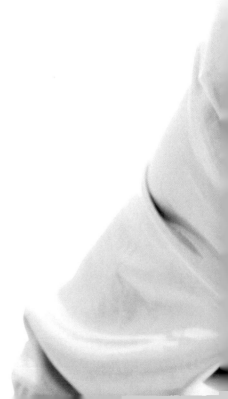

Linda Evangelista by Miles Aldridge

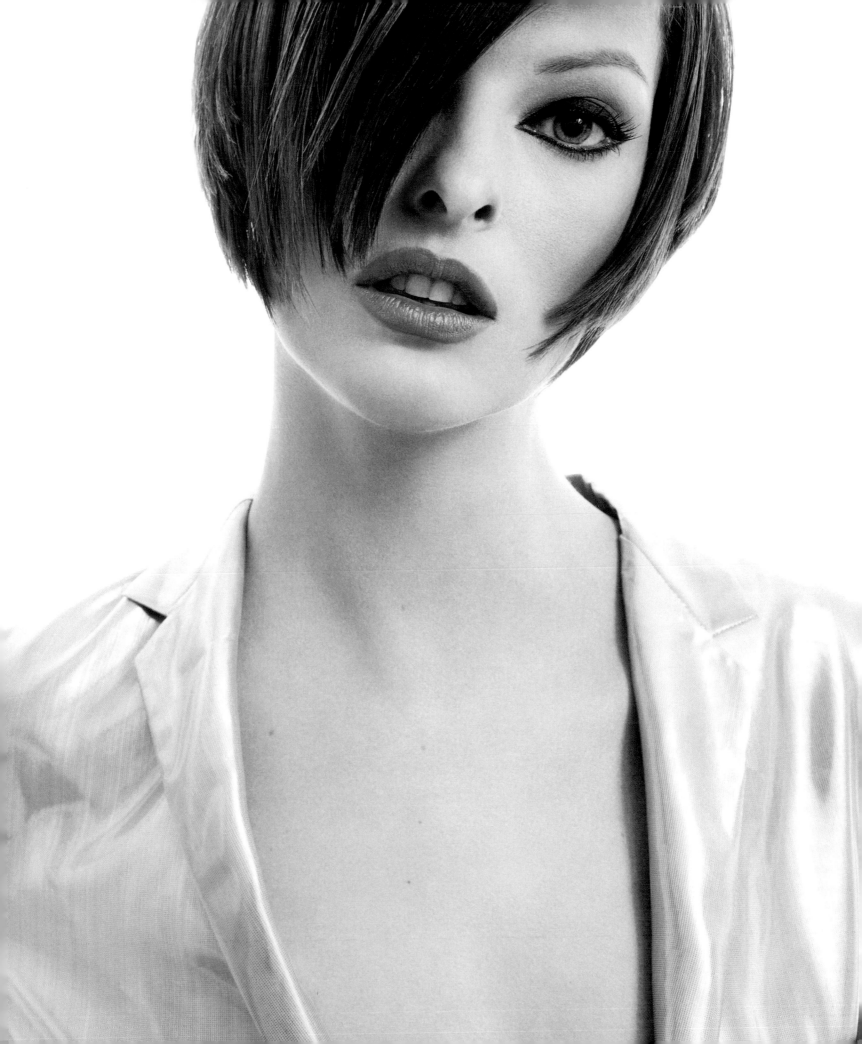

Brown Eyes

Try: Use eyeshadow or liner in gray, black, navy blue, neutral chocolate brown, or chocolate brown with a hint of red, pink-brown, gray-brown, burgundy, or eggplant. You also can use paler or medium versions of these shades as eyeshadow, as well as light mauve, light pink and peach. You can use gold shadow if your skin tone is not too sallow or yellow.

Avoid: If you have brown eyes and olive skin, skip neutral browns like khakis, taupes, and yellow-browns. They won't make your eyes look alive and will only emphasize the yellow in your skin.

Blue Eyes

Try: Use eyeshadow in fleshy pink, brown-pink, beige-pink, peachy-pink, muted mauve, grays, light dusty blues, turquoise washes, black, or all browns. Use eyeliner in gray, black, brown, navy blue, bronze-gold, or dark purple.

Avoid: If you have pink-toned skin, stay away from shadows that are pure pink. By all means, don't use strong pinks such as fuchsia, or you'll end up resembling a bunny rabbit. If you have pure blue eyes that tend not to change color, you should avoid green eyeshadow and liner. Avoid blues that are too strong because they can overwhelm your eye color.

Italian *Vogue* cover by Steven Meisel

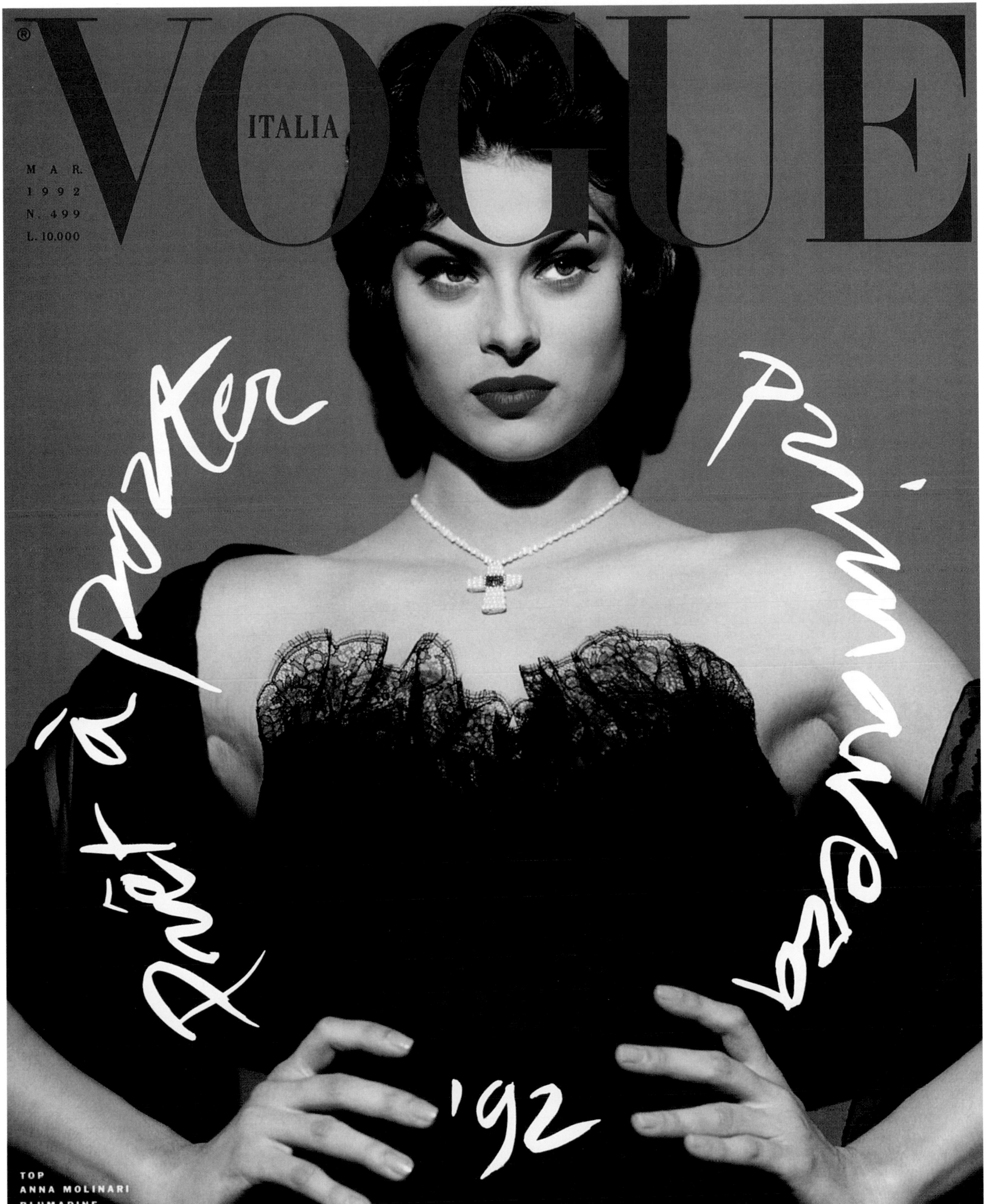
®
VOGUE
ITALIA
MAR.
1992
N. 499
L. 10.000
Prêt à porter
primavera
'92
TOP
ANNA MOLINARI
BLUMARINE

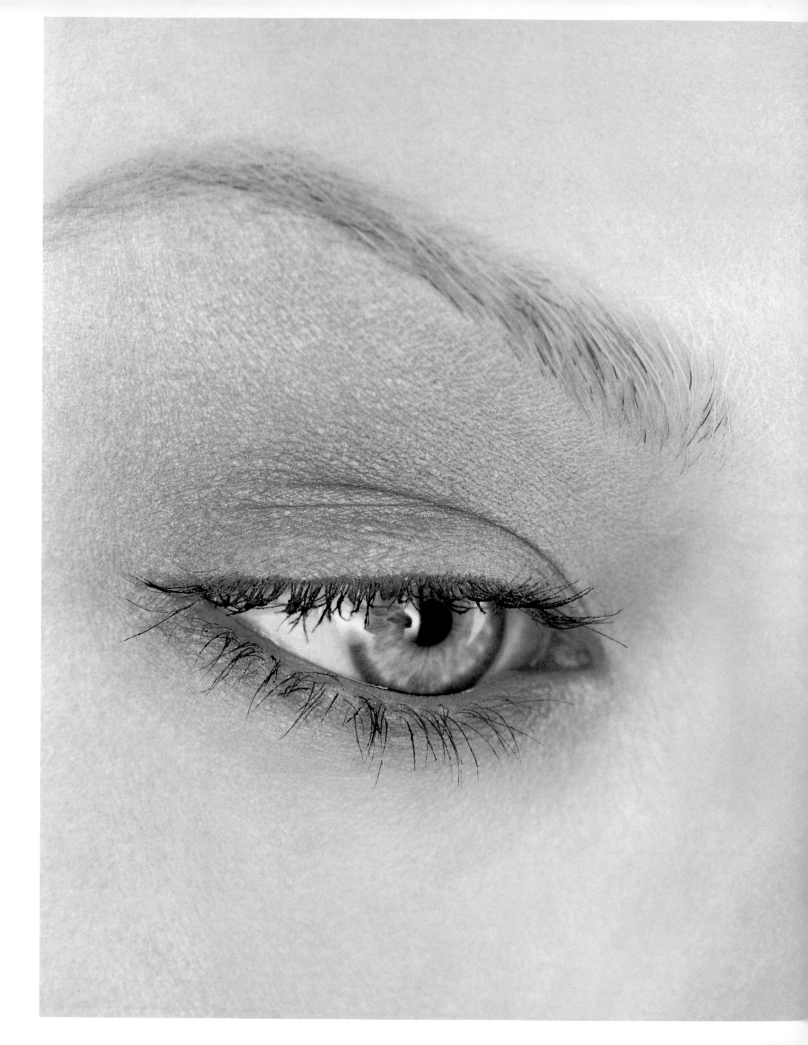

Green or Hazel Eyes

Try: Shadows in peach, light pink, muted pink, mauve, green, bronze-green, gray-green, brown-green, khaki, caramel, gold, any green mixed with gold, and all browns and grays. If your complexion is very olive and your dark circles too yellow-brown and deep, stick to the cool colors like navy blues, slate grays, mauve-grays, bright mauves, pinks, black, or eggplants. Use liner in navy, deep purple, black, gray, gold, or brown.

Avoid: Don't use any green that's not subtle. You don't want to wear bright, vivid greens because they will overwhelm your eye color. If you want to try a bright color such as teal or turquoise, make sure to apply as a subtle wash so it brightens the eye area without overwhelming your eye color.

Skip the Eye Cream

As I mentioned earlier, don't apply eye cream to your top eyelids in the morning. Nighttime is fine, but doing it in the morning will affect staying power of your eye makeup.

Previous: The beautiful combination of peachy-pink shadow and blue eyes, by Michael Thompson. Opposite: Eyes and lips by Raymond Meier

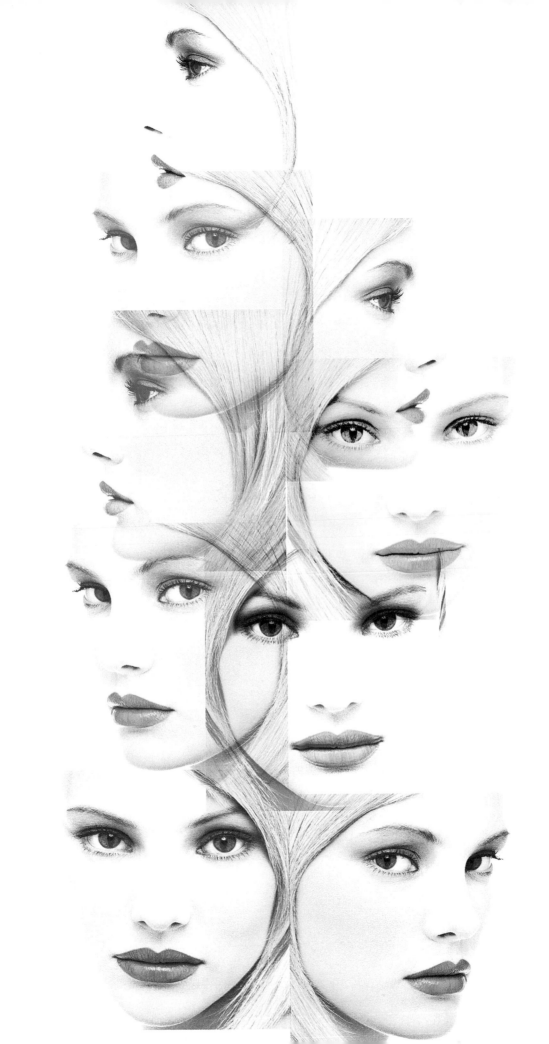

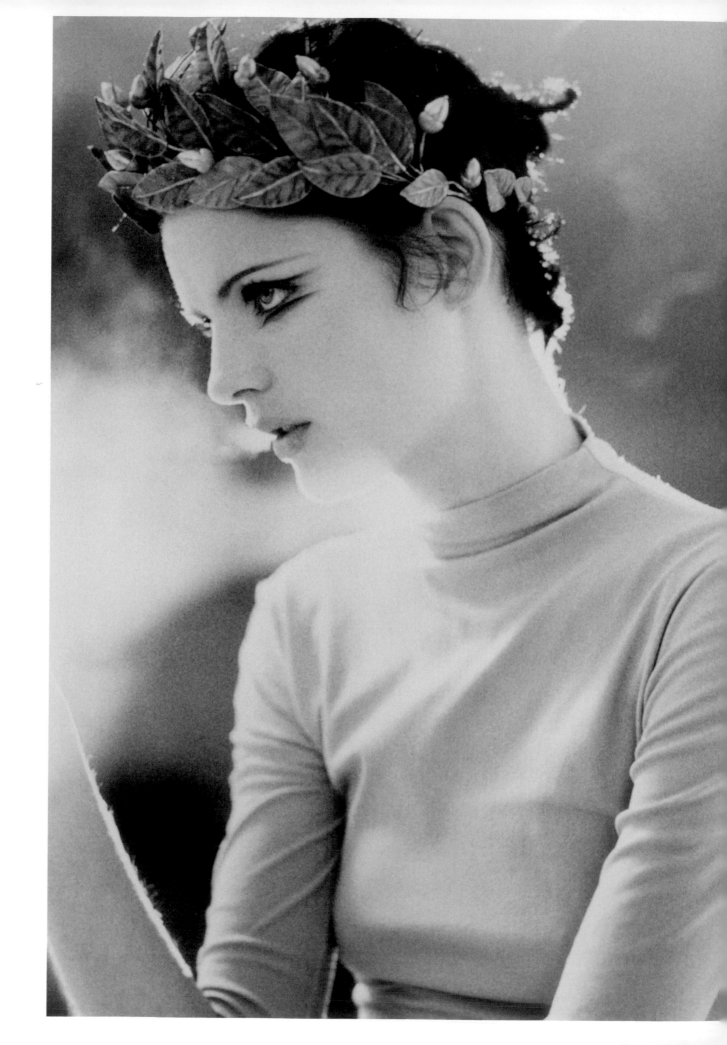

Don't be afraid to dream and experiment.

—Laura

Stella Tennant by Steve Meisel

Harper's
BAZAAR

A WHOLE NEW LOOK
MELANIE GRIFFITH,
THE DUCHESS OF YORK,
THE MAYFLOWER MADAM AND
MADONNA

Getting Started

Prime and Powder

Apply a little makeup primer to your eyelids, unless they tend to be sensitive. If you're going to apply powder eyeshadow, dust a little translucent powder on your eyelids first or after you've used primer.

Bases Covered

After you've applied primer (if you used primer on your lids), use a flesh-color eyeshadow base. I call it foundation for the lids. It has two functions. It can cancel redness, veins, and discoloration on your eyelids and serve as a base for your eye makeup so it goes on smoothly and lasts longer. It can also be worn alone for a clean, simple look.

Eyeshadow base tends to contain volatile silicones that evaporate, leaving behind a velvety finish. Use only a tiny amount; otherwise, it gets cakey and dry. You can wear powder shadow right on top of it, but I prefer to set it first with a very thin coat of translucent powder.

Bazaar cover of Madonna by Patrick Demarchelier

Cream Shadow

Eyeshadow base is different from cream eyeshadow, although the textures are similar. You can apply cream eyeshadow on top of primer, base, or both. If your cream shadow is long-wear, waterproof, or water-resistant (ask when you buy it), then you don't need to set it with translucent powder after you apply it. If it isn't, you need to set it with powder, or the cream shadow will crease. Don't set metallic cream shadow with translucent powder because you'll destroy the shine.

Wash of Color

The simplest eye makeup look is a sheer application of one color. It's like a veil of organza or silk mousseline for the eyelid. Look for eyeshadow shades reminiscent of watercolors (think Monet and his water lilies). Use an eyeshadow brush and apply a thin layer of product from your lash line to your brow bone. You want only an accent of color so you're not competing with your eye color. You shouldn't see any texture. Wear it alone or with liner and mascara.

Christy Turlington by Michael Thompson

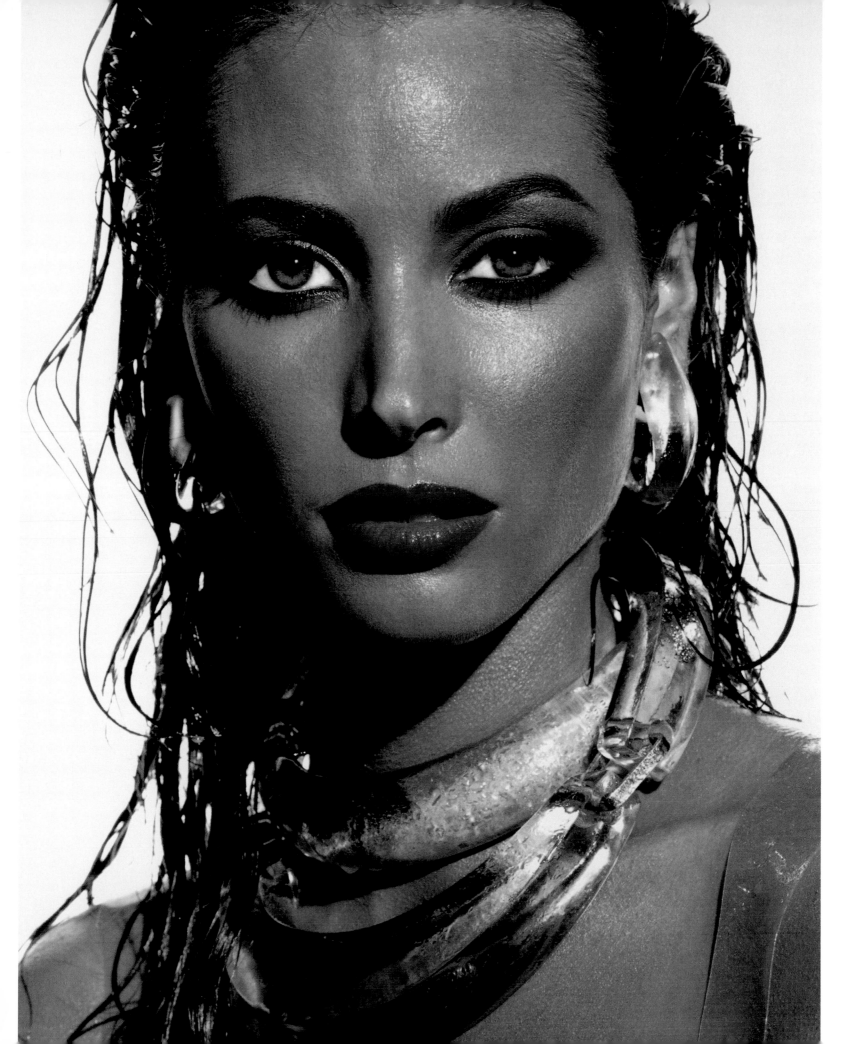

Shimmery Shadows

Highlight Your Brow Bone

A light frosty shadow on the brow bone can look a little eighties. If you like highlighting that area, stick to shadows that are light matte or slightly shimmery and transparent, not frosty, especially if your brow is low on your face. It will visually open and brighten the area.

Highlight the Inner Corner

This is a pretty look that brings a certain sparkle to your eyes, and it's a great trick for close set eyes. You can use any type of light, bright product (cream shadow, eyeshadow, or eyeliner) to bring a point of light right to the inner corners. Apply with a brush or applicator. If the product you're using is shimmery, then don't set it with powder.

Sexy Liquid or Cake Liner

Liquid or cake liner is definitely a signature look for me. I've always had a passion for that glamour eyeliner inspired by the fifties: Sophia Loren, Elizabeth Taylor, Maria Callas, Ava Gardner, and all the great beauties with their dramatically lined eyes. It always gives a sexy twist to your makeup.

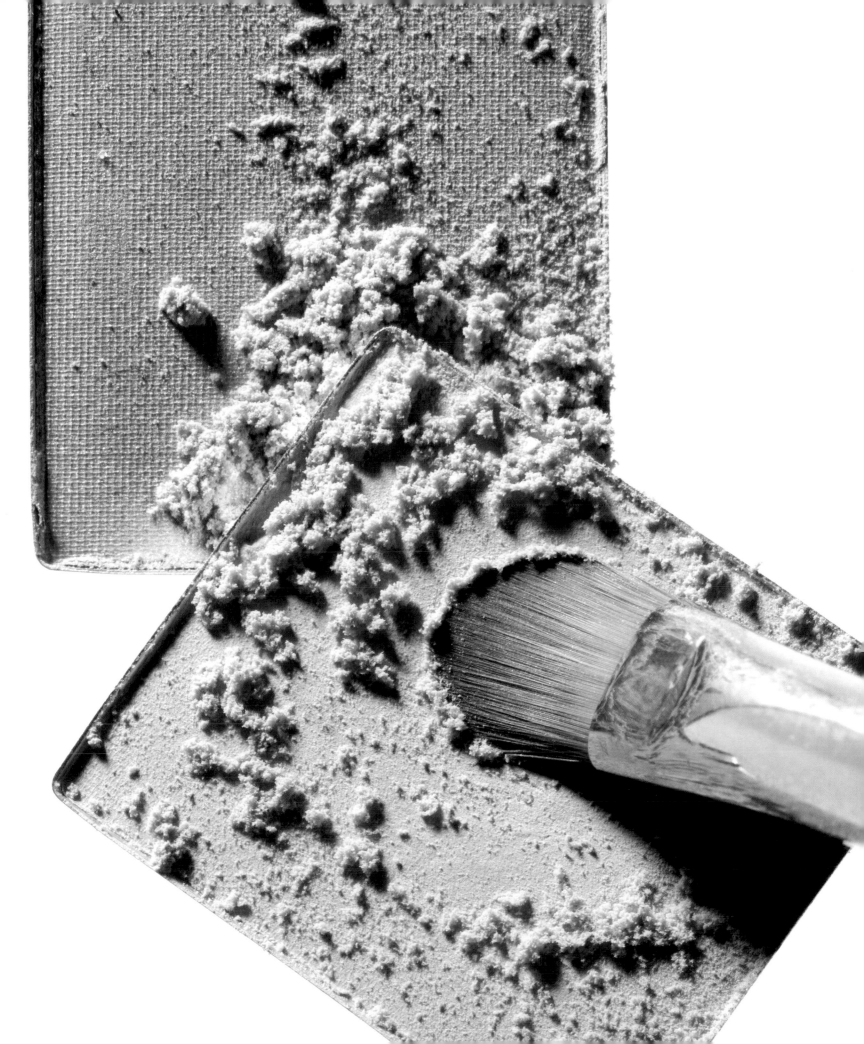

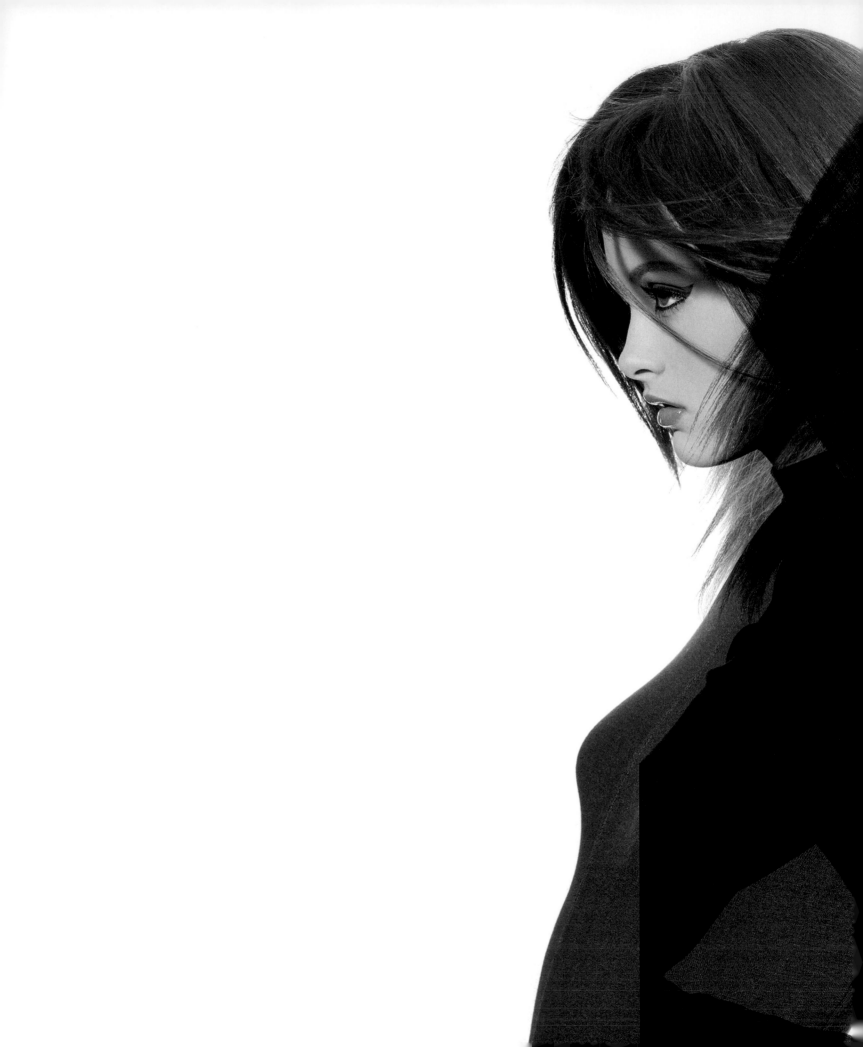

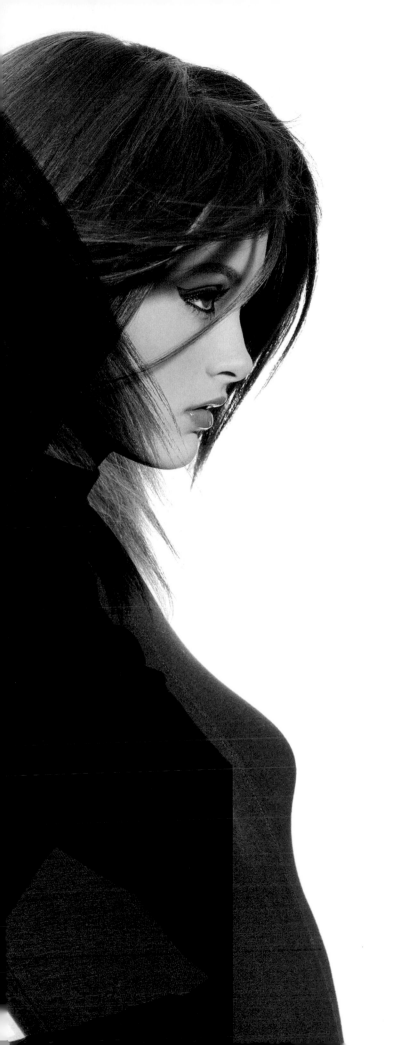

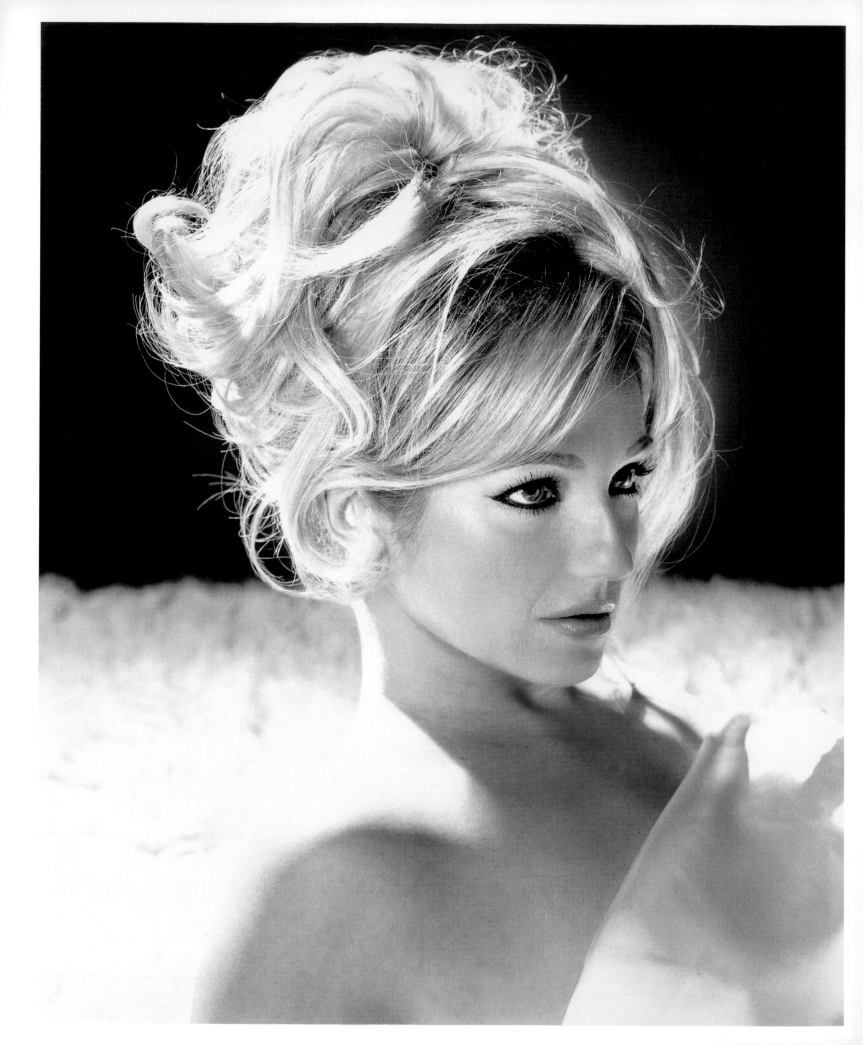

Replicating this glamorous look is not complicated, but it takes some practice getting the hang of it. The general idea is to follow the shape of the eyes (but keep in mind the eye shape rules we discussed previously). According to your eye shape and the desired look, you can thicken the liner, stretch it far out, wing it in an upward motion, or just keep it short for an accent above your lashes.

You need liquid or cake liner and an eyeliner brush that is neither too thick or too thin but very pointy. I find that liquid liners with the built-in brush or marker-like applicator have too much glide and slide to them. The cake liner has a certain resistance, so you can control the application and build up the line more easily. You can do the same look with an eyeliner pencil, but It's not going to last as long or be graphically perfect.

I rarely use cake or liquid liner under the lower lash line for real-life looks because it tends to be too harsh. What you can do is strengthen the lash line just a little with the product left on the brush. Go as close to the root of the lashes as possible. If you want a very dramatic sixties or seventies look, you can extend the liner graphically under your lower lash line.

Defining the Lash Line

One of my favorite tricks is to line right underneath the upper lash line—literally at the base and in between the lashes. This gives a beautiful definition and intensity to the lash line and looks as if you're not wearing any eyeliner. This requires a special flat, squared-off brush that you dip into your wet cake liner. Take the brush and place it right

Opposite: Ellen Barkin with sexy liner, a favorite look of mine.
Photo by Michael Thompson. Previous: Trish Goff by Raymond Meier

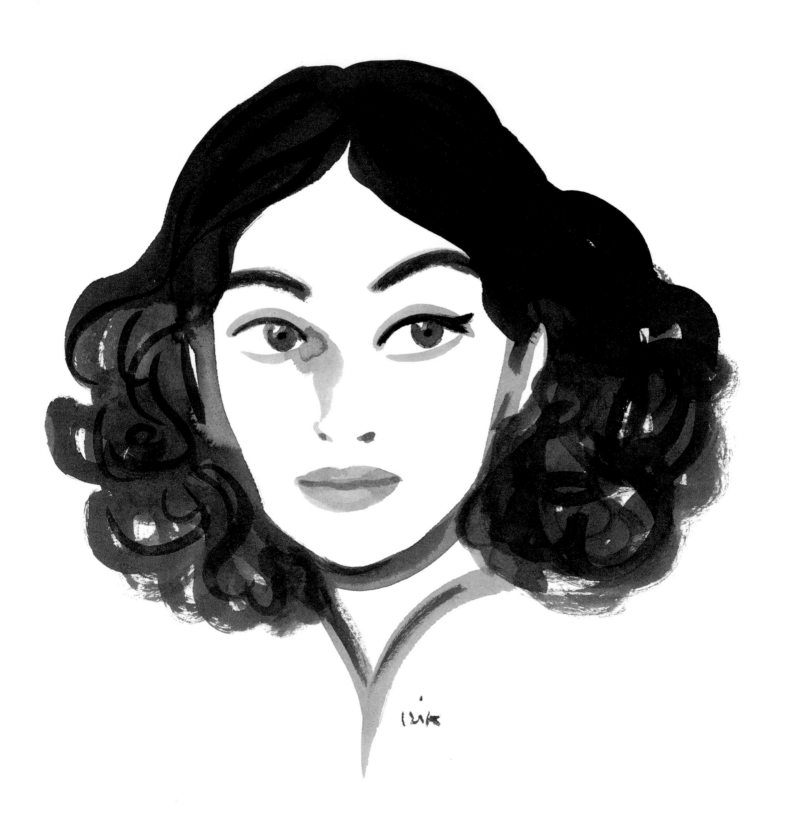

at the root of the lashes—not inside the eye—and wiggle between the roots of the lashes. Start at the center of your lash line so the most color is concentrated there. Work a little to

beauty secret > For an easy way to apply your liquid or cake liner, start with a sharpened eye pencil and sketch in the shape you want. (You can erase mistakes more easily.) Then apply the liquid or cake liner directly over the sketched-in color.

the left and a little to the right, going as far in either direction as you want or depending on your eye shape. You don't have to go all the way to either end. By building contrast right above the iris of your eye, you make the color more sparkling.

The Kohl Story

Kohl is a ground black mineral powder that has been used for centuries, mostly in African and Middle Eastern countries to protect the wearer's eyes from the sun's glare. You've seen it on renderings of Cleopatra and on countless pictures of Middle Eastern women. Because it has antibacterial qualities, it is safe to use near the inside of the eye. Today, women around the world use it for cosmetic reasons because it makes for a beautifully lined, mysterious eye. You can buy kohl powder or you can buy kohl eyeliner, but note that these products don't always contain the true kohl ingredient. Still, if you buy a kohl pencil or powder from a reputable brand, you can be assured it has been tested and approved for use around your eye area.

Sexy, retro eyeliner by Izak

beauty secret > When it comes to makeup beneath your eyes, let the makeup above your eyes be your guide. You never want to do more below than above. The idea is to have an upward effect with your eye makeup; not something that pulls attention downward. Do the makeup above your eyes first before determining what you will do below.

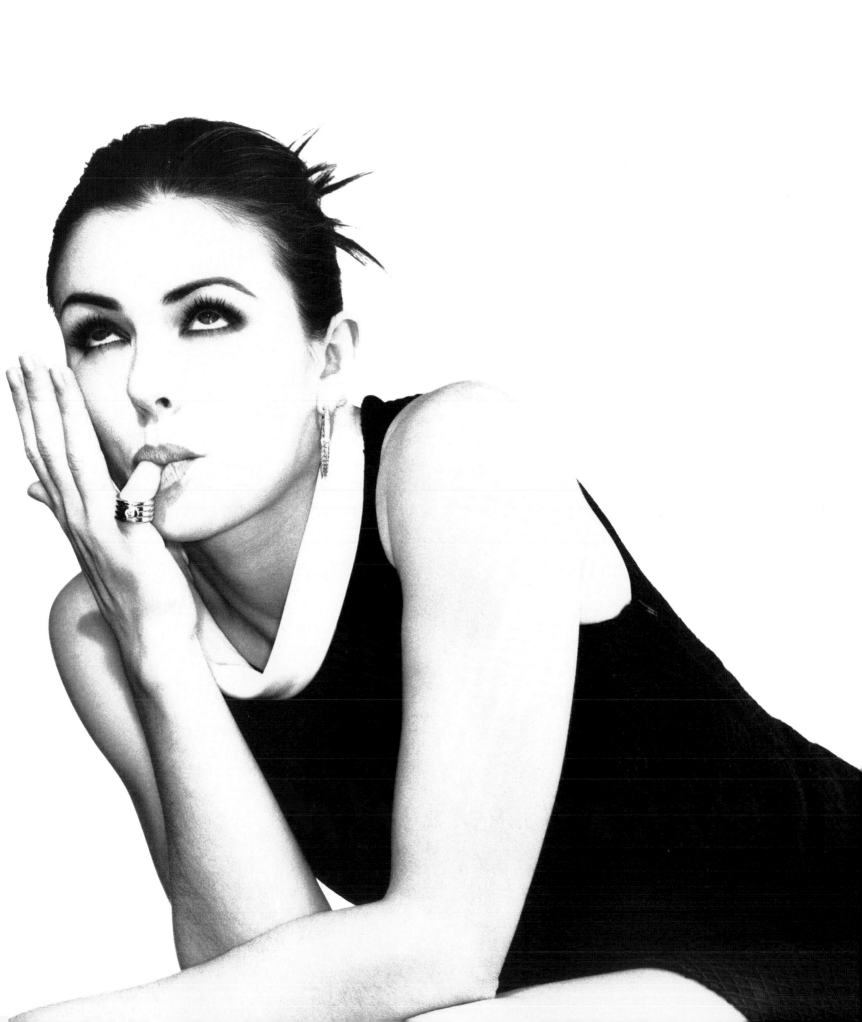

I prefer using a kohl pencil to line right inside the eyelid. If you've never done this before, it's going to take some practice because your eyes will probably well up with tears. Take your pencil (it should be sharp but not super pointy) and draw right inside the fleshy part of your eyelid. You can draw the line as light or as dark as you want, but pay attention to the eye shape rules. This is a striking look that really intensifies the whites of the eyes because it gives you so much contrast. Don't line the inside of tiny or deep set eyes because you will make them appear even smaller.

Advice for Crepey Eyelids

You don't have to avoid eye makeup if you have eyelids that have become fairly crepey and lined throughout the years. Try cream eyeshadow in matte colors. Don't use shadows that are too shimmery, pearly, or frosty because they attract attention to crepey lids. Another option is to line above or around the lash line. The idea is to keep the color and emphasis close to your iris, rather than focusing attention on your eyelid.

Curling Your Lashes

Nothing's better for adding *oomph* to straight or limp lashes than curling them. If you're one of the many women who find lash curlers scary, try a special mini-curler that does a section of lashes at a time. It's much easier to use than traditional curlers, which grab the entire lash line at once. If your eyelid and lashes don't fit the shape of the

Trish Goff times four, by Raymond Meier

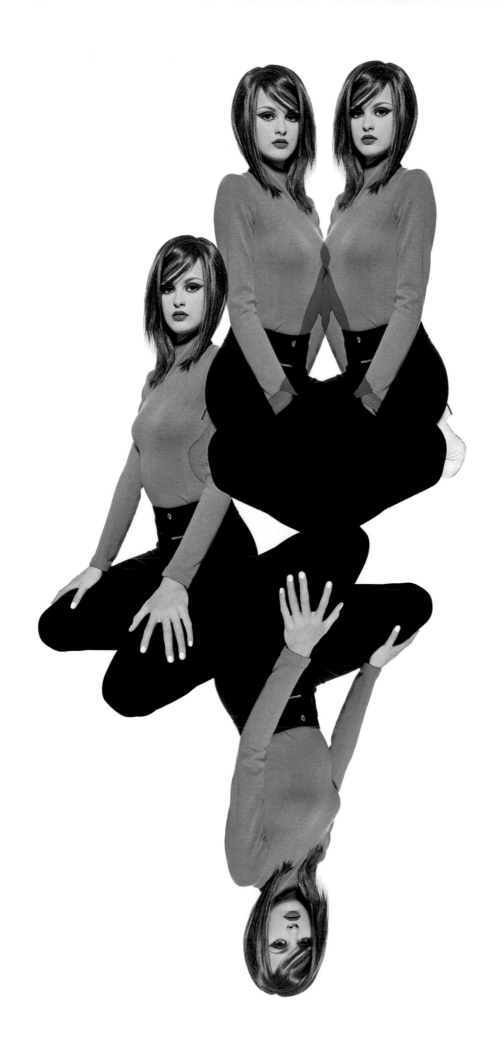

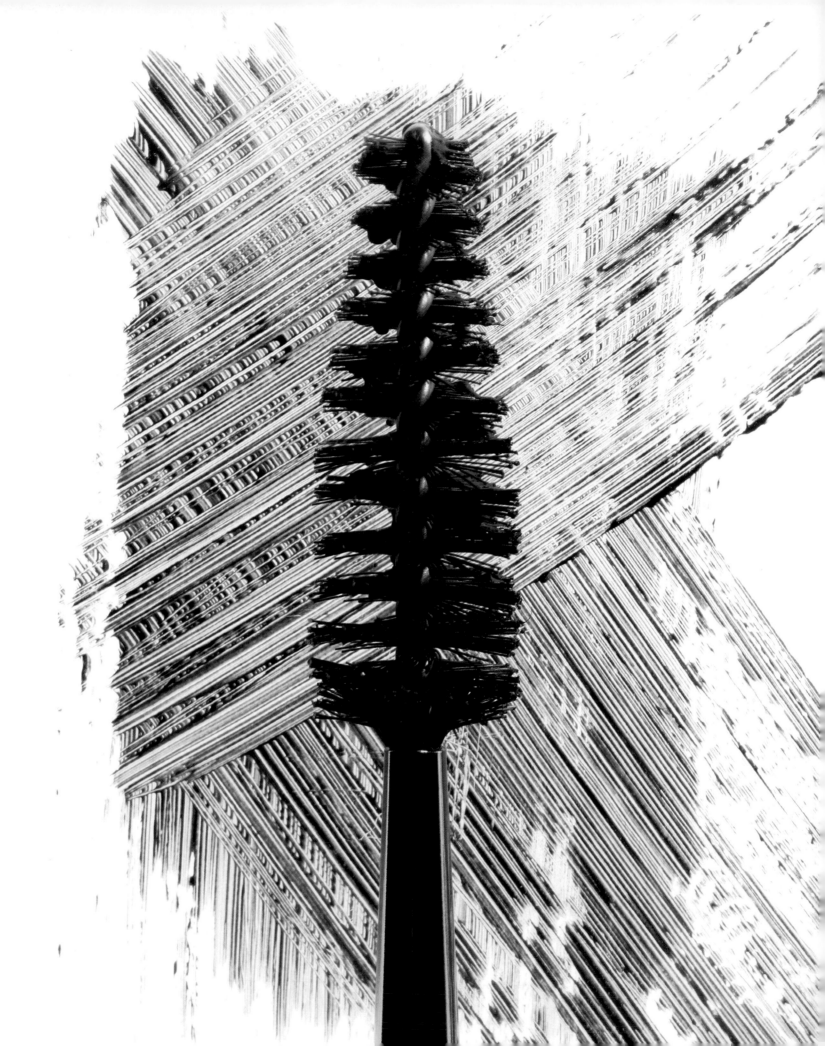

larger curler, it's almost impossible to use. Anyone can use the mini-curlers. They allow for more precision such as curling just in the center, if that's where your lashes go straight, to open the eye. Or you can curl your entire lash line to give you a young, innocent look, or the outer corners for a sexy, flirty look. You can switch between a mini-curler and a regular-size one depending on your needs.

Whichever size you use, don't abuse your lashes. If you tend to lose your lashes easily, as I do, don't curl them every day. And be careful if you curl your lashes after applying mascara because it's easy to break lashes that way.

Do You Need Lash Primer?

The purpose of these products is to thicken and elongate the lashes by leaving a white coat of primer over which you apply your mascara. (You apply it the same way you apply mascara.) If you have thin lashes, this may be the solution for you. If the primer is too heavy for your lashes and weighs them down, then skip it.

The Right Mascara for You

There are dozens of mascaras on the market, so it's difficult to know which one is perfect for you and your lashes. Throughout the years, I've learned that everyone's lashes are different, so the formula that's perfect on your friend may not be perfect for you. I've seen thick lashes, soft ones, and ones that grow downward or straight. There's

Laura loves her work and enjoys creating a look, but

she also has the ability to let you look like yourself,

which is great because I prefer to look like myself.

—Julia Roberts

Julia Roberts by Michael Thompson

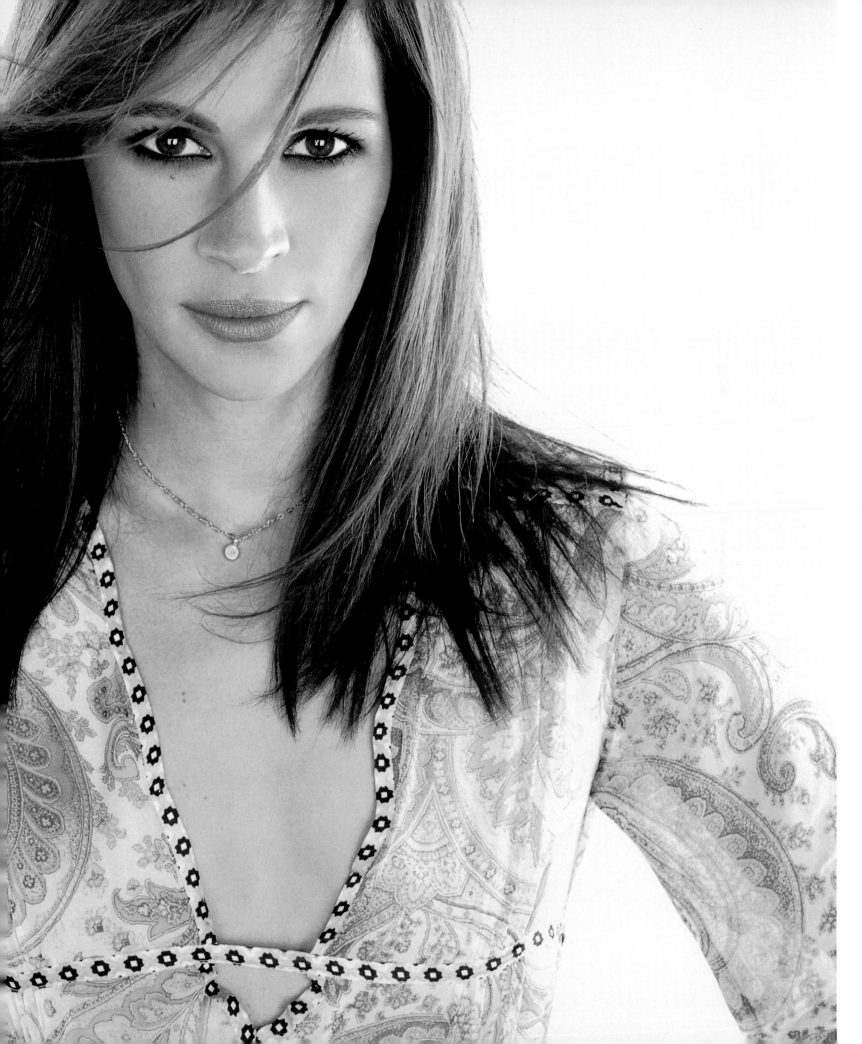

definitely a mascara out there for everyone, but you probably need to road test a few before you find the one that works best on you.

Having used every mascara on the market, and developed my own, I understand that mascara is as much about the brush as the formula. If a mascara isn't working on you, look at the brush. If it's thick and bushy, try a mascara that comes with a thinner brush or vice versa.

How to Apply Your Mascara

I like to apply mascara thickly at the base of the lash line and thin it out as I move toward the tips. I'll often use the end of the mascara brush (wipe it with a tissue to remove excess) to coat and separate the tips of the lashes. I'm not a fan of clumpy or spider leg lashes, unless that's the specific look you want. Apply as many coats as necessary. It's best to work in sections because it's almost impossible to coat all your lashes in one swoop.

It's fine to apply mascara only to the lash tips if you have allergies and can't get mascara too close to your eyes, but it can weigh down your lashes. If that happens to you, choose a thinner formula.

How to Remove Your Mascara

Don't go to bed wearing mascara! Take some good quality cotton pads, which are better than cotton balls, and saturate them with makeup remover. Press against

Inky black eyes, lashes and brows, by Raymond Meier

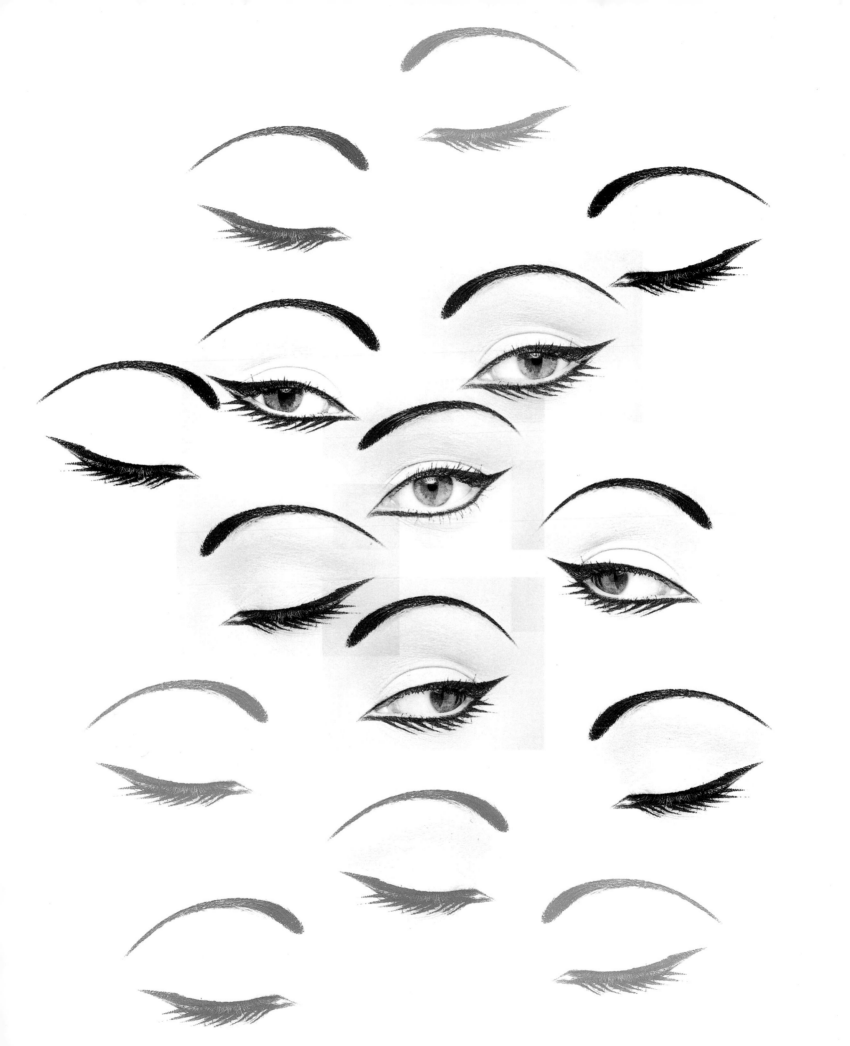

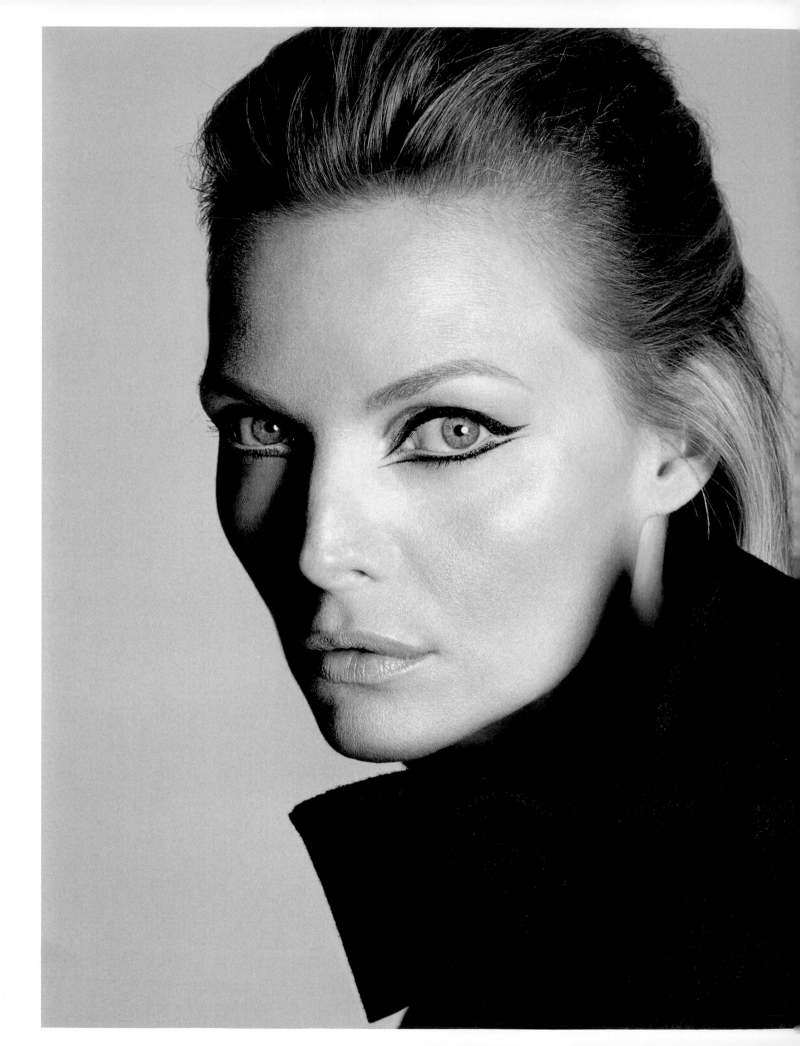

I've always had a passion for that glamour eyeliner

inspired by the fifties.

—Laura

Michelle Pfeiffer by Michael Thompson

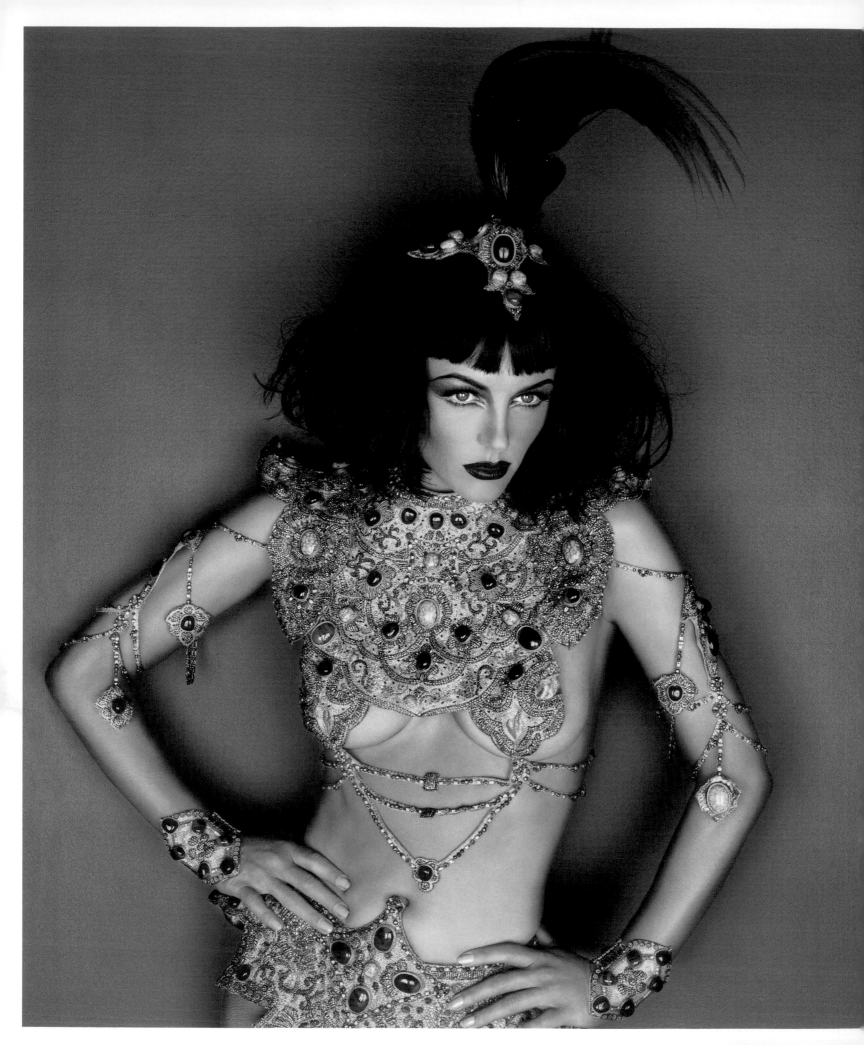

your lashes—don't rub—and use as many cotton pads as necessary. This is mandatory if you're wearing waterproof mascara. Waterproof formulas stiffen the lashes because the formulas are thick and dry. Make sure to use a remover specifically formulated for waterproof mascara. These tend to be oily, so make sure you remove the residue with water or a gentle lotion afterward.

Mascara on the Bottom Lashes

Some women believe they should never apply mascara to their bottom lashes, but it's perfectly fine to do so if you need to define your lower lashes and open up your eyes. If your lashes hit the fleshy part under your eye, you shouldn't wear regular mascara because it's going to smear. Instead, set under your lower lash line with translucent powder and use waterproof mascara on your lower lashes. Also, avoid using concealer too close to the lower lash line because the emollient nature of concealer can promote smearing.

Don't Stockpile Your Mascara

Mascara isn't meant to last more than a few months, so don't buy several at once. You need to replace it on a regular basis because of possible bacteria buildup, which isn't good for your eyes. This may sound a little silly, but when you buy your mascara, smell it. As soon as it smells different, it's time to get rid of it.

Elizabeth proves that great brows are timeless. Photo by Michael Thompson.

The right makeup can really emphasize your eye color.

—Laura

Meg, ready for her close up, by Patrick Demarchelier

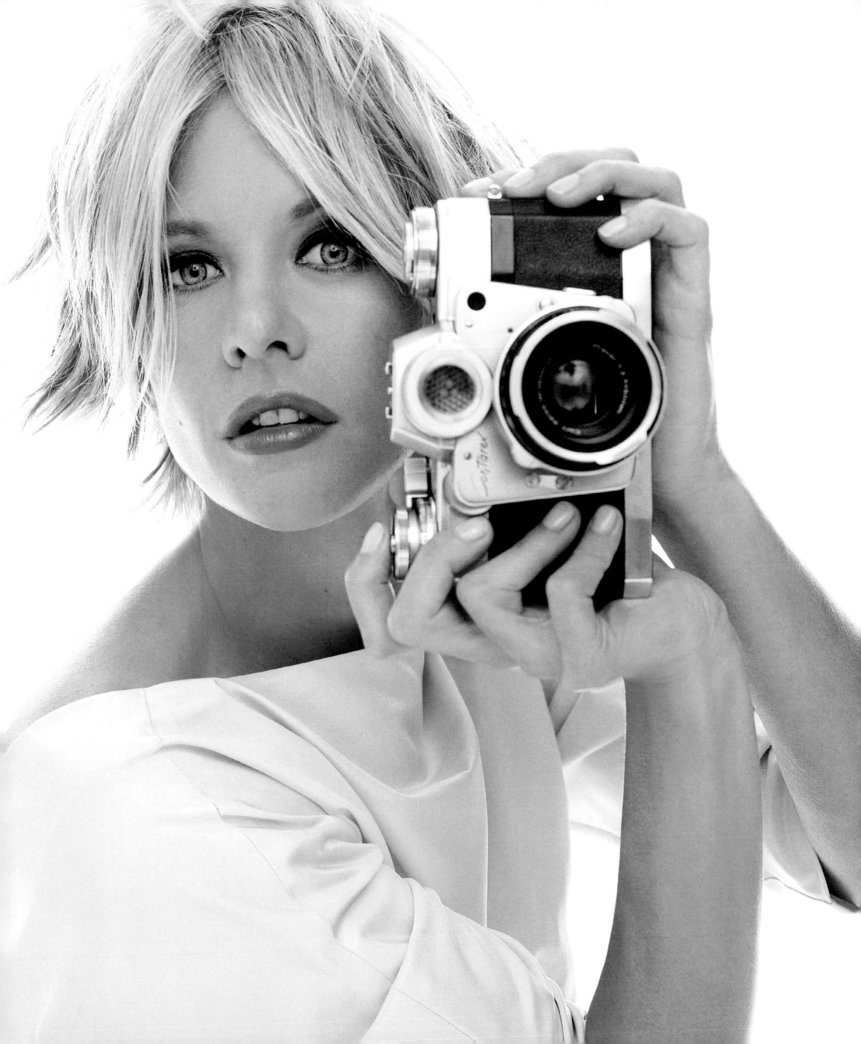

Shaping Your Brows

Getting your brows right is one of the trickiest tasks for women. It took me years before I figured out the shape that was right for me, and it was only because my friend Garren, the talented hair stylist, helped me. It's difficult to figure out for yourself. We tend to see our faces from a different perspective from how people see us. The illustrations show the most common brow mistakes and the ways to improve them. Most brow issues arise from over-plucking, so show some restraint with those tweezers. If you pluck too much for too long, the hair won't grow back. That's not an old wive's tale. It's true. Also, you should never blindly follow extreme fashion when it comes to your eyebrows. Trends by definition are meant to change, and you don't want to be stuck with a certain shape permanently!

beauty secret > If you want to lighten a dark brow, use a bit of camouflage or concealer on top. Apply very gingerly with a brush. The color will soften the darkness. The best option is to ask your hairdresser or aesthetician to lighten your brows to just the right intensity. That's the most natural choice.

Seek Out an Expert

If you're baffled by your brows, it's a smart investment to hire a good brow expert. He or she can look at your face more objectively than you can. If you can afford only one visit, pay attention during your appointment. A brow expert can shape your brows once, and then you can do the maintenance.

Correcting Your Brows

Follow these illustrations and tweeze or draw in the best brow shape for you.

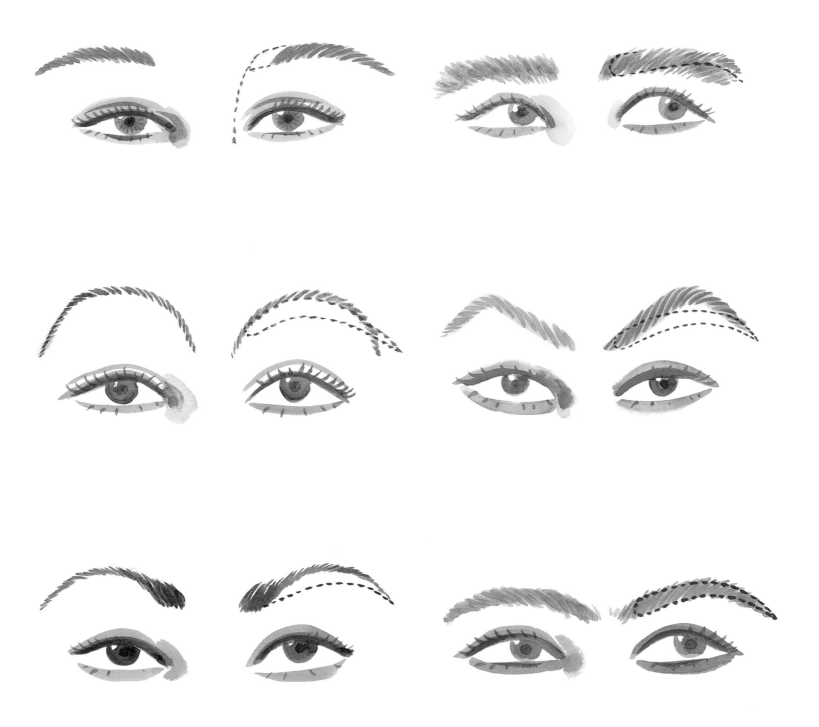

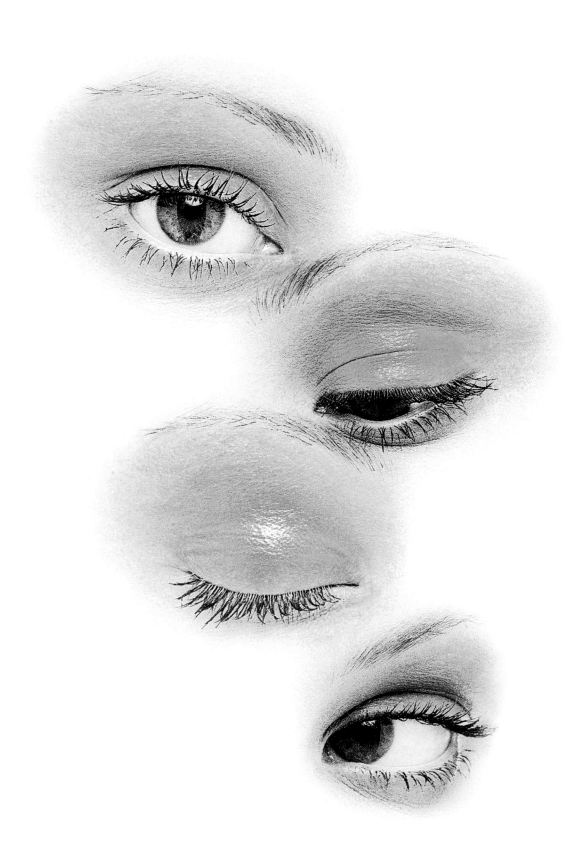

Pain-free Tweezing

I've had to pluck many models' and actresses' eyebrows throughout the years. To make it less painful, try holding a warm water compress to the area. Run a washcloth under hot (but not too hot!) water, and press it against your brow area. This opens up the pores and cuts down on the ouch factor. Afterward, you can hold an ice cube against the area to reduce pain and redness and/or apply a light antiseptic.

How to Pencil in Your Brows

Some people's eyebrows are just fine, but in general, full eyebrows are a sign of youthfulness, so consider filling in your brows with makeup if you've over-plucked. I find that brow pencil topped with brow powder is the best, longest lasting combination. The powder holds onto the wax of the pencil. Make sure to use products specially designed for your brows, and don't choose a color that's too dark. I've seen women use eye pencils and eyeshadows to fill in the sparse spots, but the colors aren't neutral enough. Good eyebrow pencils are slightly transparent and have a neutral color pigment load so they won't turn orange or reddish once you apply them.

Start your brow makeup in the very center of your eyebrow, not on the top, bottom, or inner corner. That will appear too obvious, as will a sharply drawn line. You don't want to graphically define your brow, unless that's the specific look you want.

Extreme color, by Raymond Meier

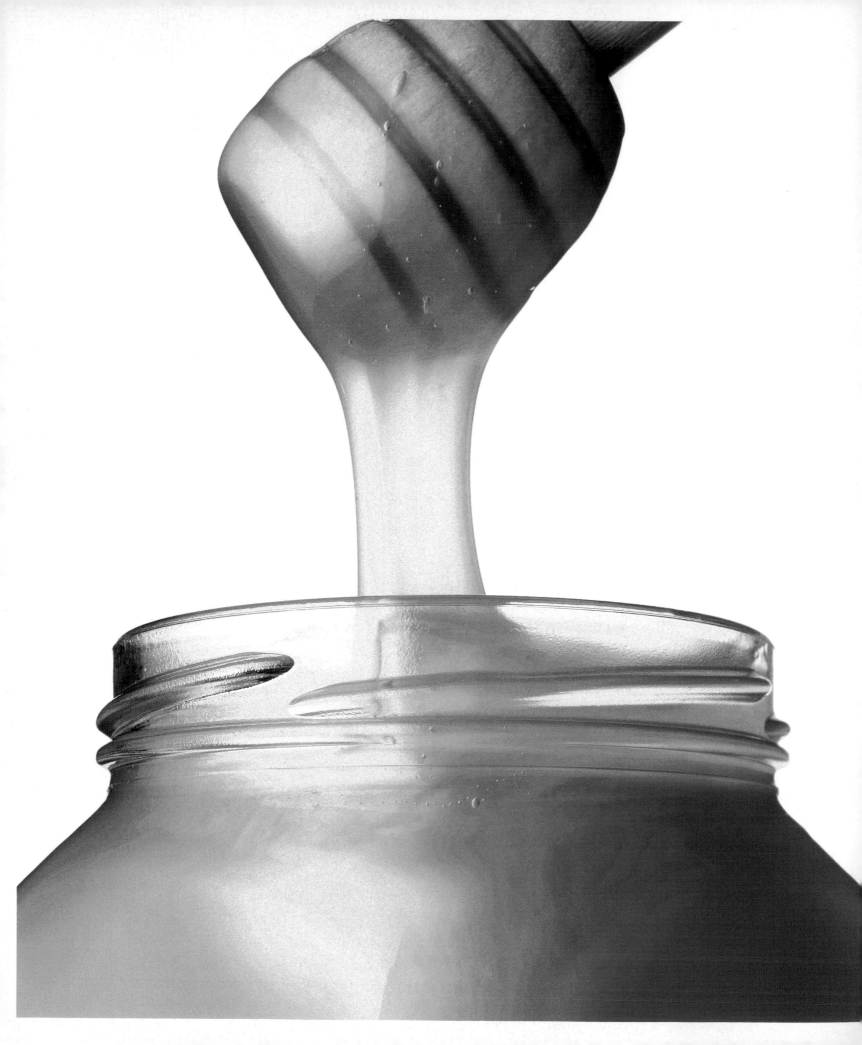

chapter nine groomed and gorgeous

I want you to close your eyes for a minute and imagine a woman who smells fabulous walking into the room. She's wearing a dress that shows off her arms and her legs, so you can tell she takes great care of her skin. She's also radiating a certain confidence and sensuality, the kind that comes when someone pampers herself with baths and nice body products. Is this woman beautiful? She smells divine, her skin looks soft, and she's giving off fabulous energy. Of course she's beautiful! And it has nothing to do with her looks or the typical definition of beauty. There are so many definitions regarding appearance, and this chapter deals with one of them: how certain beauty rituals make you look beautiful by making you feel amazing.

I'm talking about fragrance, baths, body lotions, soaps, scrubs, and candles. I'm passionate about all of these things. To me, the ability to indulge in these things is one of the best things about being a woman. Of course, that's a very French way of thinking, but the French don't have exclusive rights on it. Chances are, you love all those things too. If you don't indulge in them, perhaps you don't have the time or you never got into the habit of taking care of yourself this way. In any case, I'm going to share some of my favorite products and rituals with you so that whichever camp you find yourself in, you'll be inspired to try something new or you'll find the time to add a pampering element to your beauty routine.

Luxuriate in the Tub

I can't say enough good things about taking a bath. It's a real ritual for me, and it's been a beauty cure for centuries: from Cleopatra and her milk baths to today's

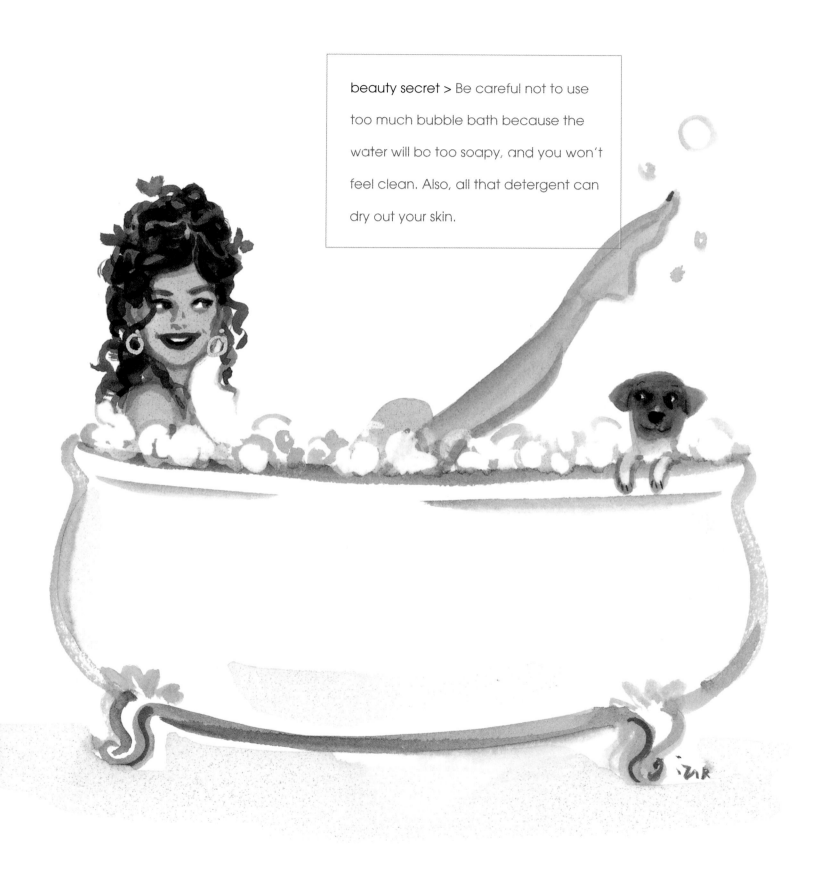

beauty secret > Be careful not to use too much bubble bath because the water will be too soapy, and you won't feel clean. Also, all that detergent can dry out your skin.

dedicated spa goers. Unless you don't have a bathtub, or you have small children who won't give you a moment's peace, everyone should be able to reserve twenty to thirty minutes once a week for a nice bath. Tell your family, partner, or roommate that you are disappearing for a little while and don't want to be bothered. This is your time to completely unwind. You're going to wash your body and wash away the stress of the day. It will be good for you and good for your relationships.

You need to do a little preparation beforehand. Make sure you have the following nearby:

Your nicest towels

Bath salts, essential oils, and/or bubble bath

A scented candle

A mat or towel for when you exit the bath

A robe

Start running the water and make sure it's the right temperature. Too cold and you won't be able to relax. Too hot and you can actually make yourself more tired. Also, very hot water can dry out your skin. The water should be warm and soothing. (Maybe you can keep a thermometer near the tub to make sure the temperature is right each time.) Next, pick something to add to the running water that you can soak in. Essential oils soften your skin, and because they have aromatherapeutic properties, they also stimulate or relax your senses. Bubble bath can be fun and fragrant, while bath salts are a good choice if you've been on your feet all day or you want to detox. After a public appearance, when I've been standing on a marble floor in a department store all day, I'll pour two cups of Epsom salt into my bath. Epsom salt is the commercial name for magnesium sulfate, which is sold in almost every drugstore for just a few dollars a carton. You'd be hard-pressed to find a better beauty bargain. Epsom salt is calming, it can help your circulation and digestion, and it has practically no fragrance so you can mix it with scented oils or bubble bath—whatever suits your mood. I also try to put something in my bath that's soothing to my skin to balance the cleansing process. A great choice is anything that contains honey, which I love because it's natural and a great skin softener. I really encourage you to create your own little recipe of products to truly customize your bathtime.

Before you slip into the tub, light a scented candle and, if you like, put on a CD of nice music or maybe even a meditation CD. Once you get into the water, just soak and relax. Don't Immediately start washing and scrubbing and shaving your legs. Save that for the final minutes. You could put on a face mask before you slip Into the tub. (This is perfect for me because I love masks, but I never have time for them.) Make an effort to put aside any concerns, stress, and problems and just focus on positive ideas. Visualize something wonderful in your mind, like a peaceful landscape or a beautiful body of water.

beauty secret > If you're going out after your bath, the scent of your bath products may linger on your body so make sure it's compatible with the fragrance you plan to wear later that night. Marry the scents that make the most sense.

Once you get into the habit of taking baths, you're going to be hooked. Even if you're restricted to fifteen minutes a week for a nice soak, so be it. Unwinding, treating your skin, and smelling some wonderful fragrances for that period of time will be very beneficial to your mind, skin, and soul.

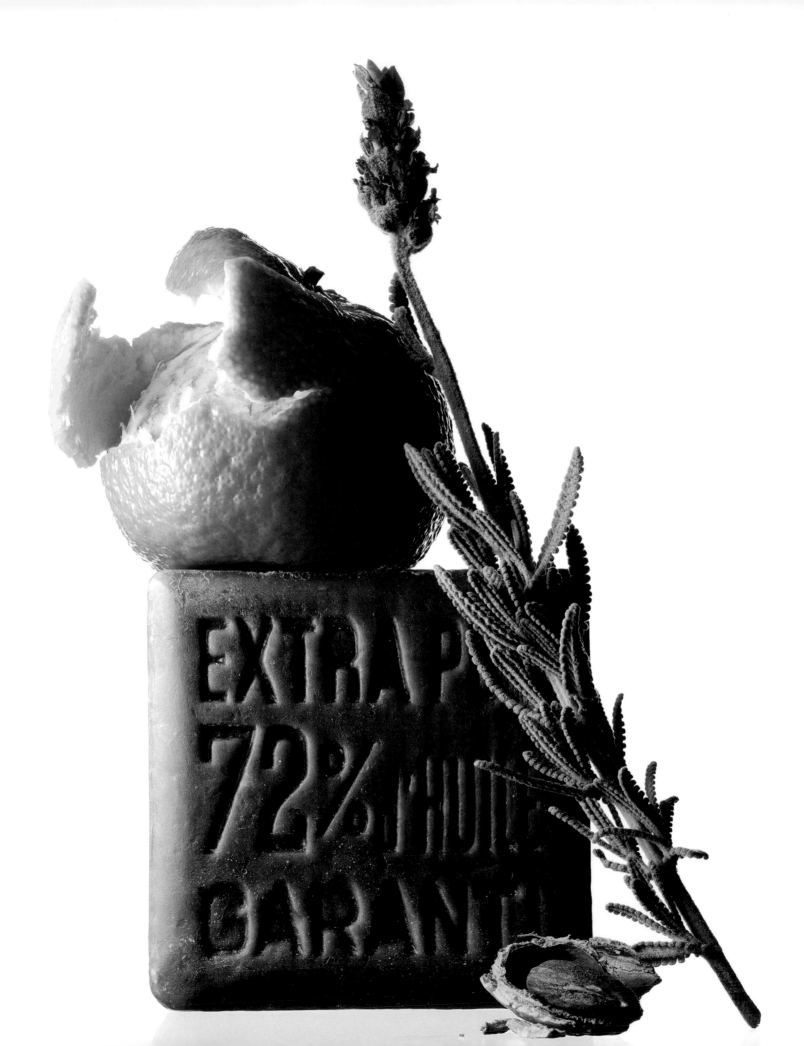

Sexy Suds

My not-so-dirty little secret? I'm completely passionate about soap: the sensuality of different soaps, the shapes, the way they foam up, how they feel on the skin. Every time I travel, I return with new bars to obsess over. Certainly, there are worse addictions to have, but mine got so bad I found myself with dozens upon dozens of bars. My supply was more than anyone, even a scrupulously clean individual, could use in a lifetime, so I gave many away. For some time now, I've been into the soaps from venerable English brands such as Penhaligon's and Floris. The scents are very sophisticated, classic, and long-lasting, and the quality of the soaps themselves are quite good. I have never liked soaps that are super artificial in terms of fragrance and color. Why would you want that on your skin?

You should look for high-quality soaps. My favorite is Marseille soap, which is cube-shaped and stamped with the words *Savon de Marseille.* Still made in the French city of Marseille, the region where I grew up, this amazing soap contains a large percentage of olive oil, which makes it wonderfully gentle and emollient. You can wash your face and body with it and it's the best thing with which to wash your delicate lingerie. Then there's my newest discovery: Alep soap, which comes from Turkey and has been made the same way for centuries. The soap is very soft and contains laurel oil. Alep soap is difficult to find, but I've tracked down a few stores in Paris that sell it. You can also find it online.

Polish Your Skin

When's the last time you gave your body a good scrub? I love scrubs because I'm so neurotic about cleanliness, but there's more to exfoliating than sloughing away dead skin cells. A good scrub also removes all the stress from my body and gets my blood pumping. If you get into the practice of exfoliating, you'll feel more in touch and in tune with your body and your skin over time.

There are so many ways to exfoliate your skin. I have a ton of scrubbing products—nylon gloves, body brushes with natural bristles, loofahs, grape seed scrubs, sugar scrubs (which I find less abrasive than salt scrubs), and even my competitors' products! Using these in the shower are my favorite way to exfoliate, as opposed to applying lotions that contain acids, such as glycolic acid, which chemically exfoliate your skin. I also prefer scrubbing in the shower to dry brushing, which is a popular technique for exfoliating and boosting circulation. With dry brushing, you take a semi-stiff body brush and rub it against your dry skin in circular motions before you get into the shower. Always scrub in the direction of your heart, so start at your feet and work your way up, and then start at your fingertips and work your way to your shoulders. Plenty of people swear by this, so perhaps it's a method you'd enjoy.

My skin is not very sensitive, so I can scrub frequently; but be careful if you have sensitive skin. Every day might be too much, and you might find that you can't scrub and shave on the same days. You definitely shouldn't use a salt scrub after you shave or else your skin will sting.

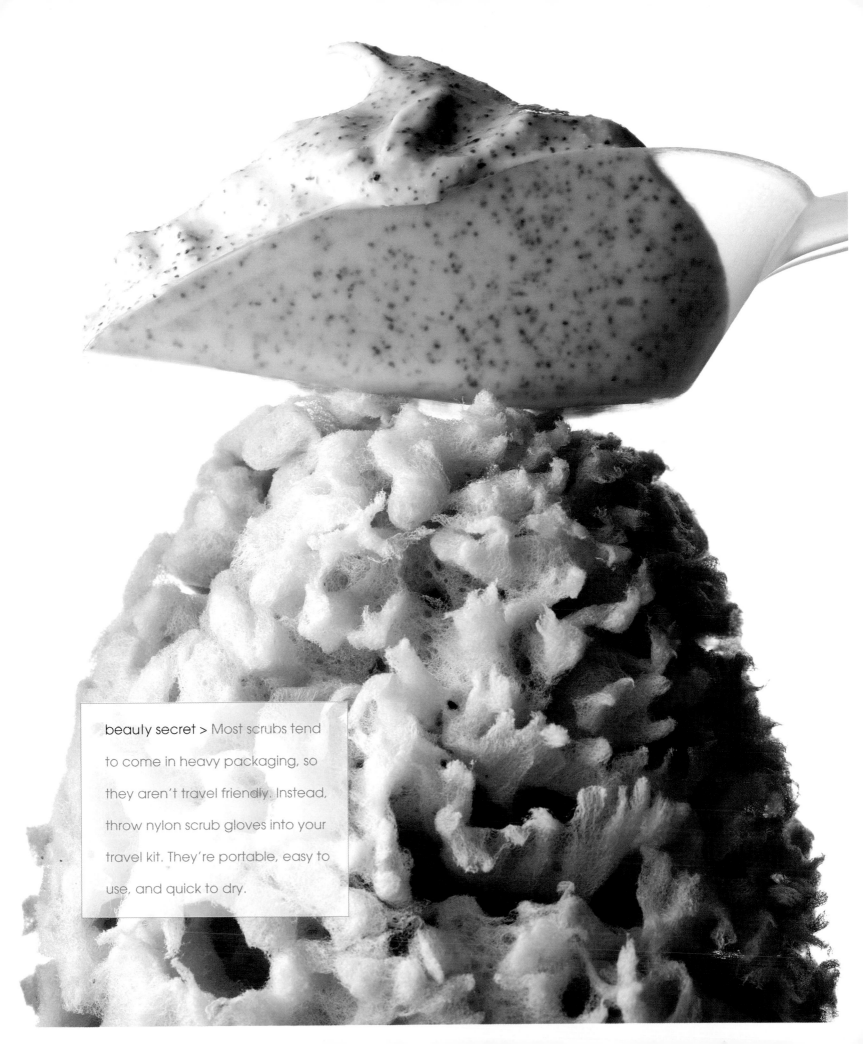

beauty secret > Most scrubs tend to come in heavy packaging, so they aren't travel friendly. Instead, throw nylon scrub gloves into your travel kit. They're portable, easy to use, and quick to dry.

Once you hop out of the shower or step out of your bath, reach for some lotion to lock in the moisture. If you've exfoliated with a scrub that contains a lot of oil, you may not feel the need for lotion, which is fine. Depending on the climate, water quality, and humidity level of where you live, plus the general condition of your skin, you're going to want to chose something lightweight or rich. Personally, I prefer lotions that do more than just moisturize. I'm a big fan of cellulite creams, which is a very French thing. I think more of those lotions are sold in France than anywhere else on the planet. Americans tend to be a bit skeptical of them. The reality is that these creams don't make you lose weight and they don't cure bad cases of cellulite, but they can help tone your skin, smooth away dimples, and improve circulation. Another option is firming creams. Look for ingredients such as ivy extract, caffeine, menthol, and camphor to really stimulate your skin.

The trick with cellulite creams is that you need to use them once or twice a day. You won't see any benefits with occasional use. I like doing what I refer to as a "cure." I use cellulite cream for a three-month period, take a few months off, and then do another three-month "cure." See how it works for you.

If you want something luxurious for your dry skin, try body oils. These smell great and the ritual of massaging them onto your skin makes you feel pampered and relaxed.

Making Sense of Scents

Growing up in Provence, I was surrounded by fields of lavender, flowers, pine trees, and herbs and learned to appreciate my gorgeously scented environment. Provence is also home to Grasse, the fragrance capital of the world because so many famous perfumes were created there. From an early age, I loved having things that smelled good on me and around me. My mother was a huge inspiration, as she always perfumed herself before an evening out with my father. It was the last phase of her pre-party beauty routine and to me, this final touch represented the height of sophistication. Her cloud of fragrance, usually the floral classic L'Air du Temps, lingered in the house before she walked out the door. She adored transparent, romantic fragrances. This ritual was not unique *chez* Mercier. It's very much part of the French culture. A woman does not go out at night unless she's securely cocooned in her favorite scent.

When I was old enough to wear fragrance, the hippie movement was in full swing. (The French term for hippie is *baba cool*.) So instead of buying classic French fragrances at the local *perfumerie,* women with their hair flowing down their backs and wearing long skirts would go to the out-of-the-way Indian shops and buy exotic scents such as patchouli, musk, and ylang ylang. When I traveled to Tunisia and Morocco, I encountered natural amber stones and learned you could rub them on your pulse points or warm spots on your body to anoint yourself with the mysterious, deep scent. I was completely seduced.

When I went to beauty school at the Carita Institute in Paris, fashion had moved onto a different degree of scent sophistication. Now I was into classic, formal Guerlain fragrances, especially Shalimar, as well as Chanel No. 19. I went back and forth between those two, but ultimately realized the scents that suited me best were those with a warm, sweet, powdery base. Today, I wear fragrance all the time, even when I'm working in my garden. I change my scents according to my mood, the season, the location, the climate, and the occasion.

If you had to describe your relationship to scent, what would it be? Do you have a signature scent? Even though it's an old-fashioned concept, I find it incredibly sexy. Just like a makeup signature, such as Paloma Picasso's bright red lips, having an identifiable scent is a way to enhance and proclaim your personality. Women always ask me how to find a signature scent and the only answer is through trial and error. You'll know what scent marries best with your skin! You'll miss the scent when you're not wearing it and when you do wear it, people will compliment you on how fabulous you smell.

Aside from a signature scent, there are ways to make a fragrance distinctly yours. You can layer two or more different scents, which I prefer; I used to mix rose and amber, my signature scent for years. You can also layer fragranced body lotion with your favorite scent.

beauty secret > There are three different concentrations of fragrance: perfume, which is the strongest and has the highest concentration of fragrance oils; eau de parfum, which is in the middle; and eau de toilette, which is the lightest.
The lighter concentrations can be worn day or night, while perfume is best reserved for nighttime use. You never want to be too aggressive with your scent.

Beauty by Candlelight

Candles are a great way to fragrance your home and add a decorative touch here and there. The best candles tend to be expensive because of the quality of the raw ingredients, like the wax, fragrance, and wick. You can get the most out of them by following a few tips:

1 Before you light your candle, trim the wick. A short wick ensures that the candle will burn cleanly and evenly. Before you relight a candle, take a tissue and break off the burned part of the wick.

2 Don't overdo it with candles because you can irritate your sinuses and overwhelm your sense of smell. You don't need three candles in every room. One will suffice, and blow it out at some point. The scent will continue to linger.

3 Don't mix scented candles when their fragrances oppose each other. When you have a sophisticated candle, you want the pure scent of it. However, scents such as rose and jasmine are beautiful in combination.

4 Be smart about the candles you burn during a dinner party. It's fine to burn a candle in the kitchen while you're cooking, as long as the scent is not overwhelming or perfumy. Don't burn a scented candle while you're eating because it will interfere with your guests' senses of smell and taste in regards to the food. It's ok during dessert, however, especially if the candle is a dessert-inspired scent.

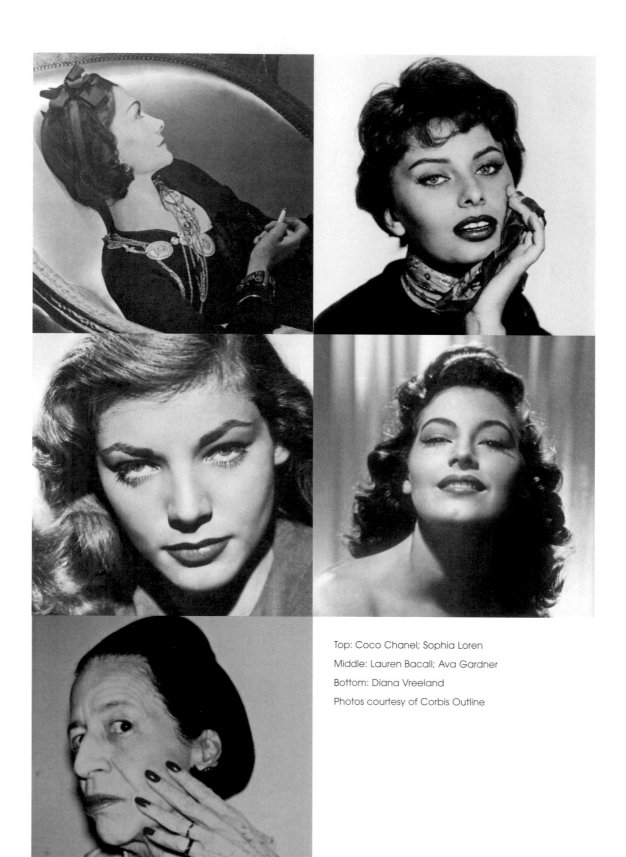

Top: Coco Chanel; Sophia Loren

Middle: Lauren Bacall; Ava Gardner

Bottom: Diana Vreeland

Photos courtesy of Corbis Outline

chapter ten my beauty icons

The women in this chapter have inspired me immensely. It's not the fact that they're world-renowned beauties—it's that each possesses a huge amount of character in her face. Examine them closely and you won't find perfect noses, mouths, eyes, and chins, but rather an assemblage of interesting, often imperfect parts that makes them so memorable. These women truly made the most of their looks and helped me to appreciate what makes a face unique.

Ava Gardner

When MGM executives came across a small-town studio photograph of a then-unknown Ava Gardner, they saw a big-time Hollywood star. They knew her long, flowing, wavy hair, arched eyebrows, and cleft chin could seduce audiences. When you look closely, you notice her eyelids were a bit heavy, which gave her face a sense of mystery and wit, making her even more unforgettable.

Anna Magnani

Anna Magnani's earthy appeal and poetic features set her worlds apart from her contemporaries. A star of Italian neorealist cinema, the actress captivated both European and stateside audiences with her wide-set eyes, soulful gaze, and "skin the color of Devonshire cream," as Tennessee Williams put it. For me, she is proof that strong character can raise one's beauty to an unexpected level. She symbolizes the perfect mix of a confident earthy nature, deep sensuality, and intellectualism.

Sophia Loren

With her hourglass shape and wide, sensual mouth, Sophia Loren is all woman all the time. Never coy about her sex appeal, the Italian actress famously announced that she owed her curvy, va-va-va-voom figure to spaghetti. Her appetite for life, her down-to-earth nature, and her elegant attitude make her irresistible. Amazingly, when she started acting, she was criticized for having hips that were too wide and a nose that was too long. Can you imagine her in *Man of La Mancha* or her other movies without that magnificent figure and proud nose? Her signature makeup has influenced me for years and, despite changing times and trends, her image never fails to inspire me.

Katharine Hepburn

Hollywood didn't know what hit it when Kate Hepburn entered the picture. Her strong bone structure and cool, angled features should have warned them: This invulnerable, confident beauty used her intelligence and tomboyish style to become one of film's grandest dames.

Maria Callas

Known as "La Divina," Maria Callas won international fame for her impressive vocal range. But her look was just as impressive—heavy brows; Cleopatra-like, flared eyeliner; and painted-on vermilion lipstick that gave new meaning to the term stage makeup. She was the perfect atypical beauty—grandiose and gorgeous at the same time!

Diana Vreeland

The hyperbolic editor became the stuff of legend with her grand style decrees "Pink is the navy blue of India," she said, and for launching the careers of offbeat beauties. When she believed in something, she followed through with it the whole way. By donning shoe polish black hair, rouged cheeks and earlobes, and a ring of scarlet lipstick, Vreeland herself became the visual embodiment of her all-or-nothing philosophy. At the end of the day, her amazing sense of style overshadowed the fact that she, as she put it, had the face of a cigar store wooden Indian statue.

Greta Garbo

They called her "The Face." Sculptural, mysterious, and a little sad, the actress's legendary visage hypnotized moviegoers only to leave them wanting more—the elusive, intensely private Garbo held a world of secrets behind her sleepy eyes. Proof

Clockwise from top left, Anna Magnani, Katharine Hepburn, Barbra Streisand, and Greta Garbo

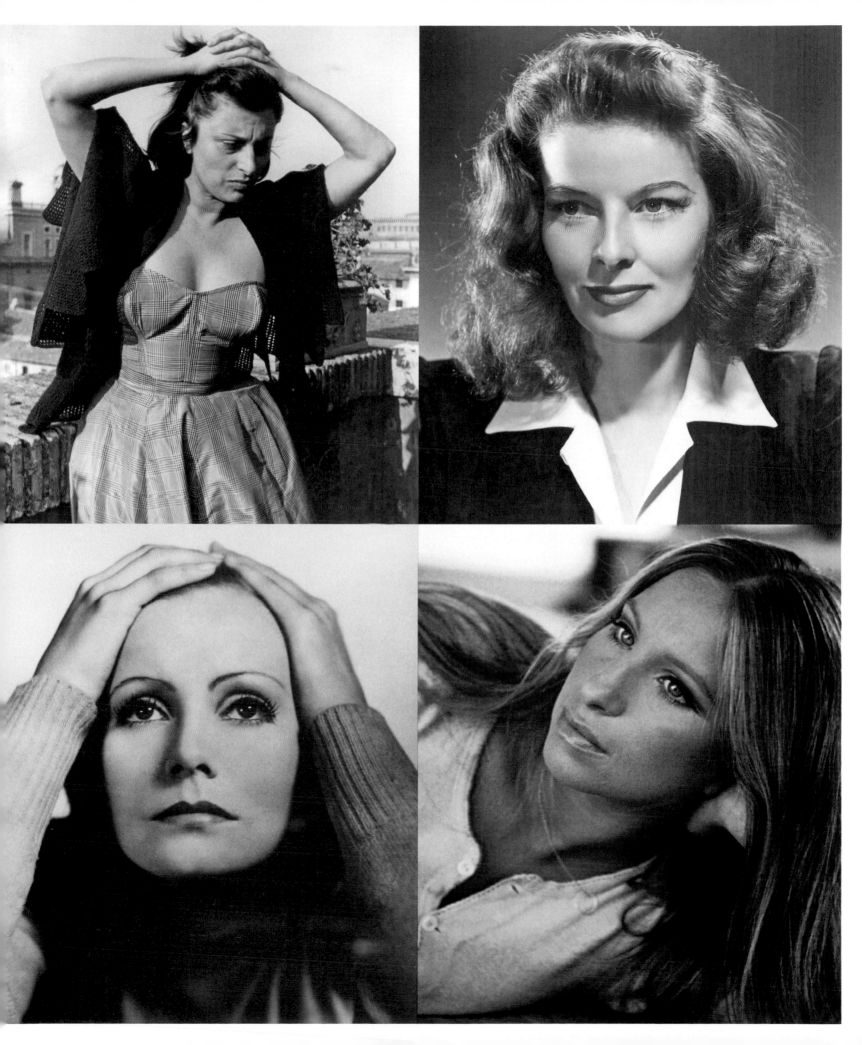

that the public is still under her spell, the United States, as well as her native country, Sweden, issued a postage stamp with her portrait last year. Look at any image of her, and you can see how she used makeup and lighting to craft a personality.

Barbra Streisand

"I arrived in Hollywood without having my nose fixed, my teeth capped, or my name changed," said Barbra Streisand. "That is very gratifying to me." Not to mention to her notoriously devoted fans, who find her integrity as inspiring as her iconic profile, elegantly lined eyes, and immaculate manicure. What does this tell you? When you fall under the spell of her beautiful voice, you're not thinking of her nose or her makeup, just a magnificent character.

Lauren Bacall

In her early days, Lauren Bacall's classic blonde beauty landed her one modeling gig after another with style bible *Harper's Bazaar*. However, it was her sexy, wise-beyond-her-years eyes that had moviemakers clamoring to put her in their films. Even the quickest glance from underneath those heavy lids rendered men powerless and earned the actress the nickname "The Look." Women who have heavy eyes like Bacall's should think about the mysterious gaze they posess. What expression they can project!

Audrey Hepburn

With her diminutive figure, quirky smile, and liquid-lined doe eyes, Audrey Hepburn became America's sweetheart, eclipsing the luscious vixens before her. She didn't need the bells and whistles of her bosomy predecessors, either; an elegant flick of inky black liner, a fringe of short bangs, and a tidy ponytail constituted Hepburn's style: the holy grail of taste-seeking women today. But look closely! Her nose had a prominent presence on her face that a modern day actress might be tempted to change. Would you dare change it?

Paloma Picasso

Few understand the efficiency of bold color and graphic form as well as jewelry designer Paloma Picasso. The silver slashes of X's and elegant scribbles that character-ize her jewelry, not to mention her bold stamp of red lipstick, have become her calling cards and are recognized around the world. And what a coincidence that her angular profile serves as a reminder of her father's Cubist inclinations.

Coco Chanel

The gold-chained quilted handbag, the tweed suit, Chanel No. 5, the two-toned shoes, and so on: Coco Chanel was a self-made woman and a self-made beauty who

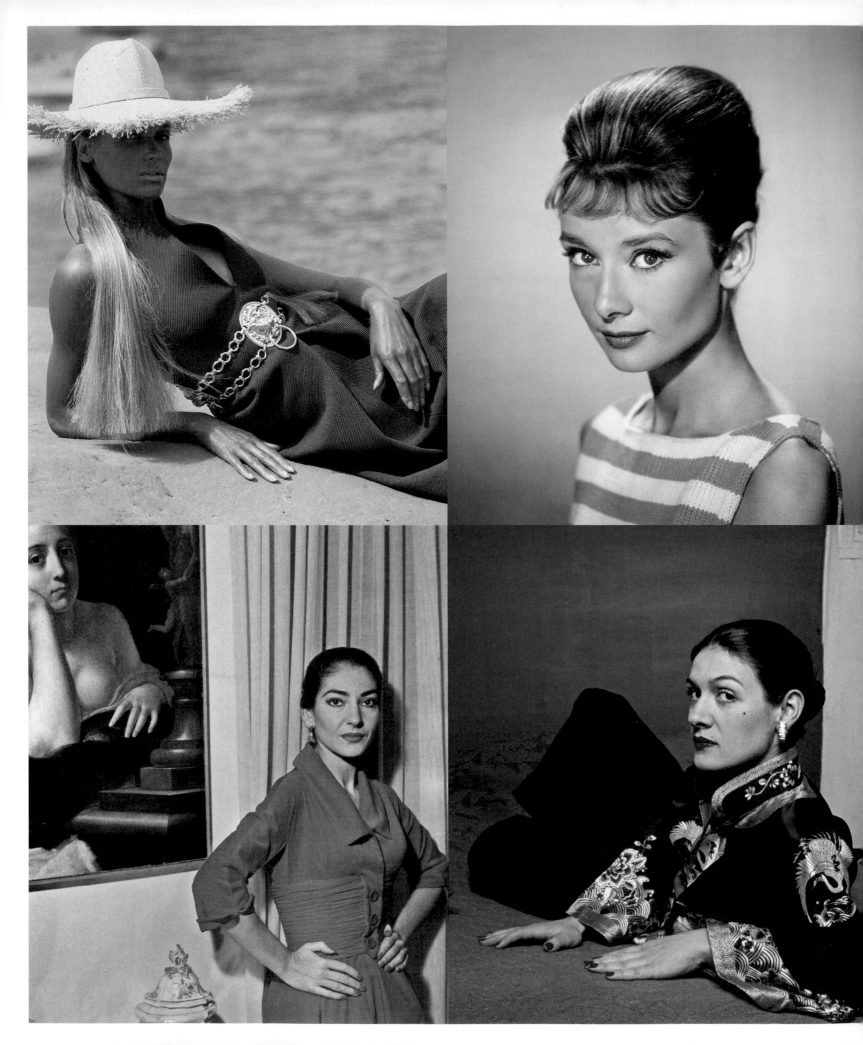

helped define luxury, style, and a ladylike appearance for generations. Her commitment to presenting women as elegant, modern, and privileged is still heavily felt today. When you see pictures of Chanel close up, you may see that she was far from a traditional beauty, so to speak; but her personality combined with her style made her look unforgettable.

Veruschka

Long before models' long-limbed, saucer-eyed, otherworldly stare became the standard, sixties supermodel Veruschka was giving good face to top shutterbugs such as David Bailey and Richard Avedon. Her great talent, far-set eyes, and statuesque figure afforded her the ability to transform into any character through edgy makeup and styling, which brought a rush of new energy to a once tame field.

Clockwise from top left, Veruschka, Audrey Hepburn, Paloma Picasso, and Maria Callas

acknowledgments

Merci beaucoup to the following people:

My Danielle and my talented Serge Normant for their unconditional love and support. My longtime friend and makeup teacher Thibault Vabre who opened the door for me. My parents who encouraged my career and my sister Sylvie and Jean Philippe and my nieces Emilie and Vanessa. My friend Madeleine Cofano who believed in me even through hard times.

My PR people Marcy Engelman and Dana Gidney for their ongoing support. Kerry Diamond for her professional collaboration, hard work, and talent. Izak Zenou for his incomparable style and warm personality. Ranee Flynn for her longtime friendship and immense talent. Sandra Collado and Julian Peploe for their exceptional work and dedication. Judith Curr and Greer Hendricks at Atria Books for appreciating my message and philosophy. Hannah Morrill at Atria Books for her dedication.

Marc Hispard for his encouragement and for giving me the opportunity to come to the United States. You're a delight to work with.

Madonna by Patrick Demarchelier

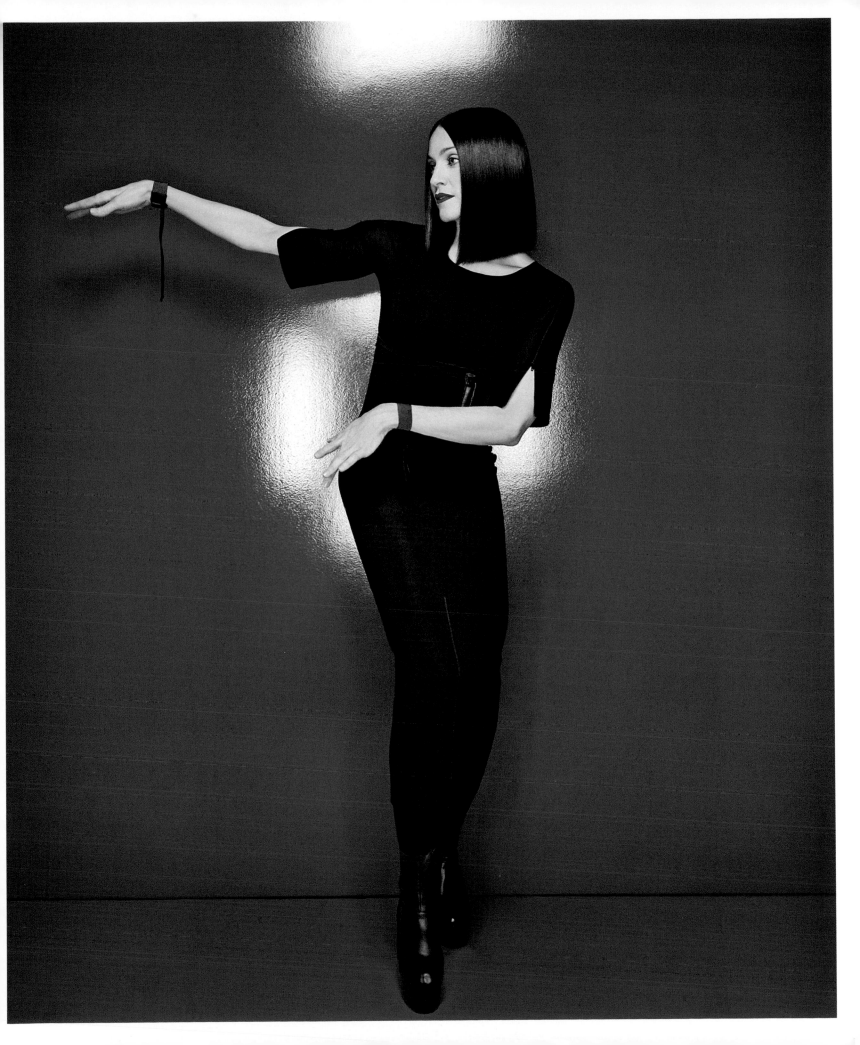

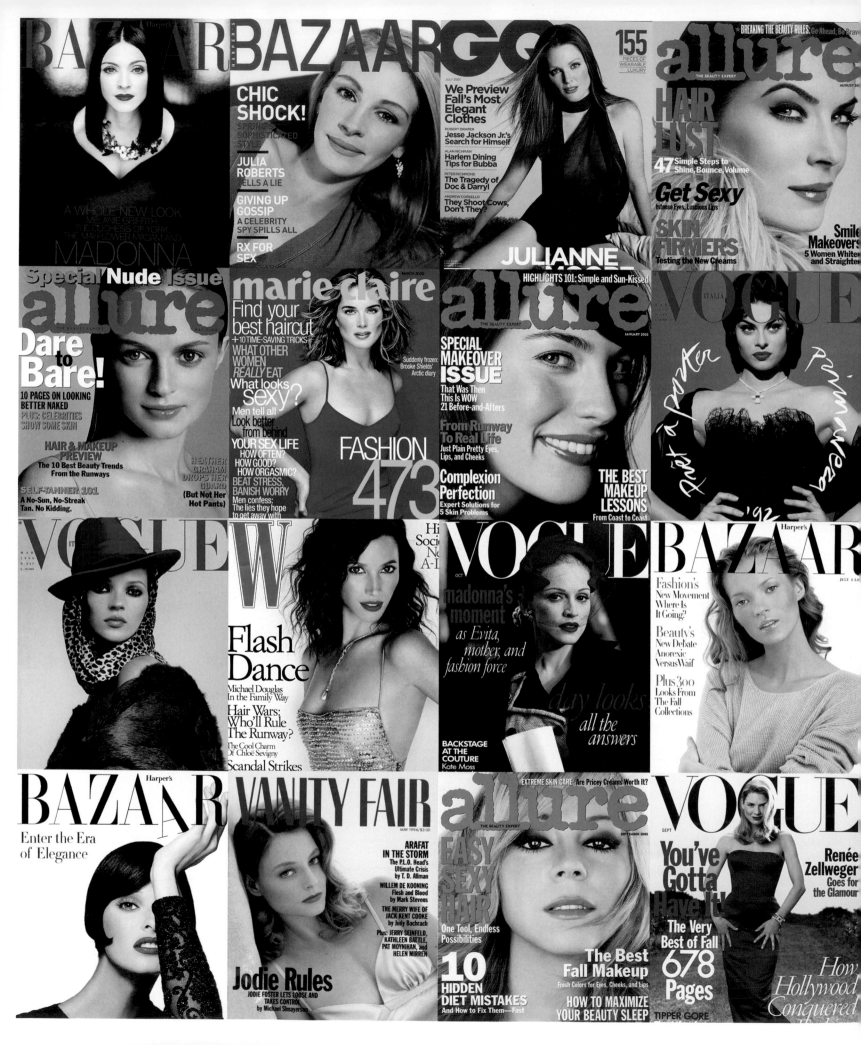

Brigitte Lacombe for her gracious participation. Patrick Demarchelier for his exceptionally generous collaboration in this book. Steven Meisel for his incredible talent, love, and belief in me. I've learned so much from you! Thank you for your help with this book. Michael Thompson for his patience despite my crazy schedule and his kindness, generosity, collaboration, and trust. Gilles Bensimon, Peter Lindbergh, Sante D'Orazio, Bruce Weber, Ellen von Unwerth, Paolo Roversi, Toscani, Walter Chin, Steven Klein, Irving Penn, Sarah Moon, Richard Avedon, Raymond Meier, Miles Aldridge, Andre Rau, and all the other photographers I've worked with over the past twenty-six years.

Allure's editor in chief Linda Wells, *Glamour*'s Felicia Milewicz, and all the other beauty editors who have been so supportive throughout the years. Liz Tilberis, whose vision and beauty I will always admire. Carlene Cerf for her impeccable taste, honesty, and friendship and for introducing me to Steven Meisel. Paul Cavaco for his talent, kindness, and dedication. I love you. The talented and inspiring Kevyn Aucoin, Francois Nars, Pat McGrath, and Stephane Marais. Odile Gilbert, Sam McKnight, Orlando Pita, Guillaume Bérard, Bruno Pittini, Julien d'Ys, Oribe, and the other hairstylists whose beautiful work appears in this book. All the very special, dedicated people at the Laura Mercier

Company, including my amazing international sales force, organized and supportive Houston-based corporate staff, and exceptional national and regional artists. Special thanks to Janet Gurwitch for giving me the opportunity to realize a dream, Sharon Collier for her trust and professionalism through the years of building Laura Mercier Cosmetics, and Carlene Gregg Victor for her loyalty and for teaching me everything at the lab and beyond.

Madonna—needless to say, I'll always love you. Mariah Carey—thank you for the exceptional experience, kindness, and trust. Celine Dion—you're a delight to work with! Julia Roberts—thank you for your ongoing love and trust. Sarah Jessica Parker—what to say?! Your friendship and appreciation give me the warmth in my heart one always needs. Julianne Moore, Ellen Barkin, Jennifer Lopez, Susan Sarandon, Angelina Jolie, and all the other women with whom I've worked for their trust and loyalty and for helping me love my job more than I thought possible. Linda Evangelista and Christy Turlington—we had golden years together, didn't we? Oprah Winfrey for her appreciation and all the opportunities she has given me. Thanks for being who you are.

Tom and Garren for their talent, friendship, and support always. Isabella Rossellini for her kind collaboration and precious friendship. Bruce and Sophie Nadell for their friendship, professional help, and true loyalty. Loren Plotkin for his friendship and protection. My close entourage of faithful friends: Cathy Bodart, Danielle Lefranc, Veronique de Villele, Julien Bubera, Jacky, Steve, Patty, Babette, Annie Siegel, Damiano, and Thierry, Pascaline, and Victoire Gineste. And lastly, to Peter Reznik for giving me a new life.

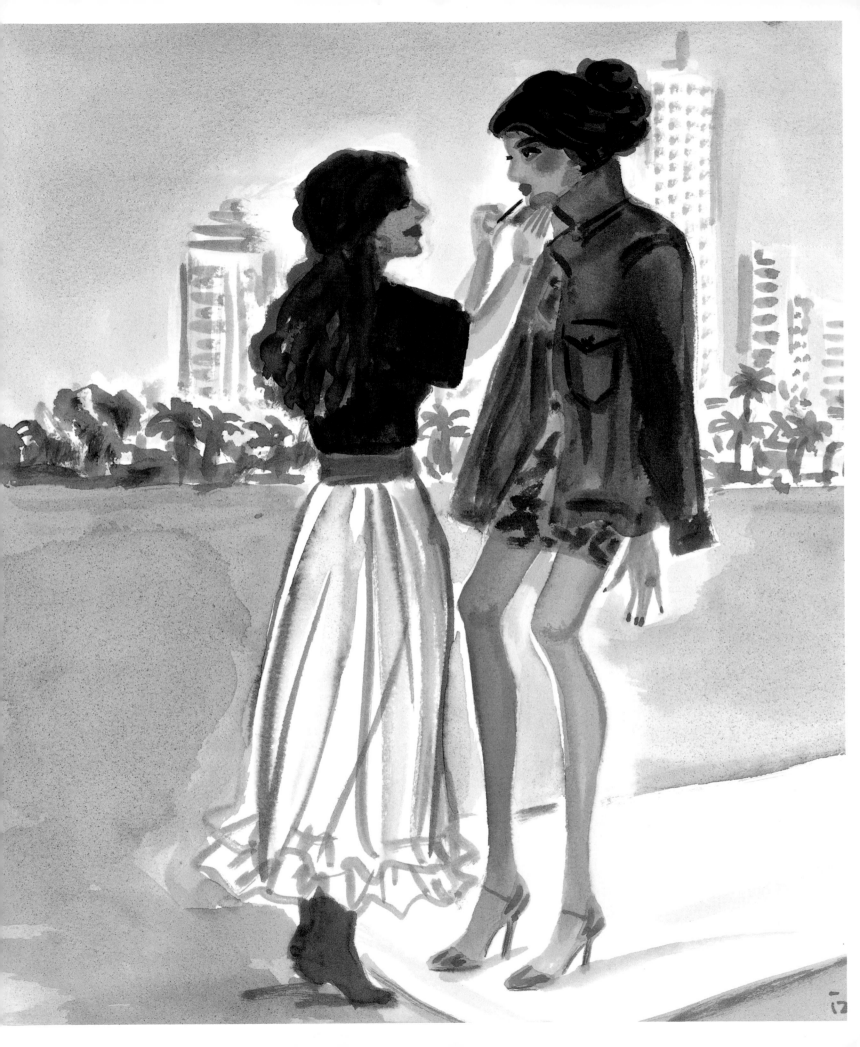

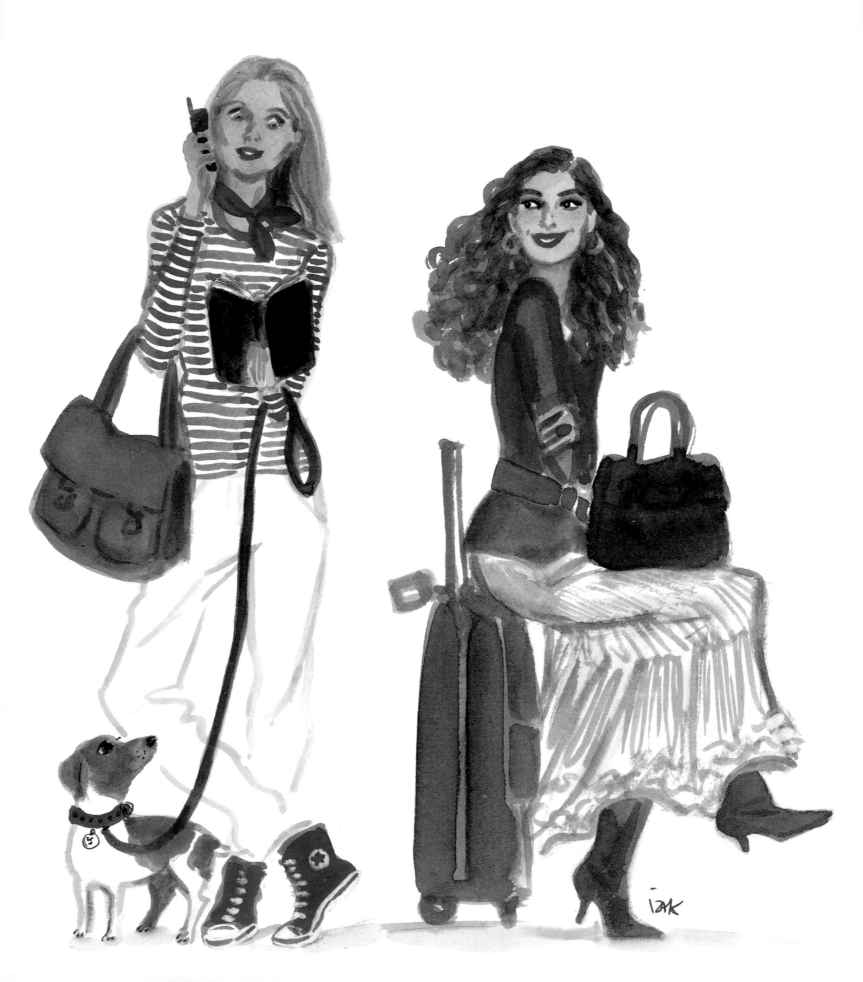

Credits

Cover and pages 3, 4, 7, 11, 90, 106, 128, 131, 148, 149, 150, 155, 156, 157, 180, 199, 205, 231, and 235: Izak. Page ii, 122, 154, 167, 176, 185, 191, and 200: Raymond Meier.

Page iv, xvi, 27, 57, 120, 141, 170, 197, 227, and 228: Patrick Demarchelier. Page x, 47, 112, 135, 142, 163, 168, and 228: Steven Meisel. Page xii: Silvia Mautner. Page xiv, 12, 15, 28, 39, 43, 44, 48, 58, 68, 71, 76, 78, 82, 88, 97, 100, 105, 111, 126, 137, 152, 164, 173, 178, 183, 189, 192, 194, and 228: Michael Thompson. Page xviii: photos courtesy of Laura Mercier. Page 24, 31, 32, 35, 36, 62, 64, 67, 87, 92, 95, 116, 119, 138, 144, 147, 158, 175, 186, 202, 208, and 211: Richard Pierce. Page 40: Patric Shaw. Pages 52 and 75: Laspata DeCaro. Page 81 and 161: Miles Aldridge. Page 98 and 125: Sante D'Orazio. Page 102: Glen Luchford. Page 109: Albert Watson. Page 151: Marc Hispard. Page 216, 221, 224, and 224: photos courtesy of Corbis Outline.